CONTENTS

The Big Weight Is Over

How to Achieve Sustainable Weight Loss through Progressive Resistance Training

By

Gavin Turnbull

Copyright Page © 2020 by Gavin Turnbull

INTRODUCTION

For most of us keeping our weight at a level that protects our health and keeps us active can prove quite difficult. Especially during these modern times with time saving devices, the automation of labour-intensive tasks, desk jobs and the easy availability of processed foods. A combination that can lead to a more sedentary lifestyle and a constant calorific surplus, hence weight gain.

With weight loss being a desirable goal for most, a whole market has evolved, and we constantly see organisations offering weight loss plans, slimming club memberships etc. And they all work to a degree, but they tend to have one thing in common and that is that they are not sustainable without a high degree of eating discipline. For most us its' that constant need in the discipline of watching our food intake that results in the success falling by the wayside. We naturally don't like feeling hungry. Diets are only ever a temporary way to weight loss, where as resistance training offers a permanent solution.

Also, by sticking to a strict low-calorie diet you can end up losing muscle as well as fat and that results in a lower metabolism. You become skinny fat. That's why people often find that their weight goes back on even quicker when they relax the discipline. You end up Yo-Yo dieting. How many of us have constantly gone through that cycle?

If you're reading this, then like me you're probably in your or approaching your mature years and looking for a solution that doesn't involve strict diets or hours and hours of cardio exercise. Most of us are. Albeit this advice works for anyone. The younger you start, the easier it is to achieve the results and maintain them.

However, before you go any further, let's make something clear:

You can't out train a bad diet!

You can't maintain weight loss if you're never active!

I never said it would be easy. With pogressive resistance training you must be in it for the long term, albeit for most people you only need to commit 3-4 hours per week of training. And the good news is unlike dieting you get to eat a normal amount of food for your height and weight and in some cases more. Hopefully, this book explains how progressive resistance training works in the simplest of terms, by explaining some of the science behind it and the exercise regime required in about 2.5 – 3 hours' worth of reading. So, no rambling on like other books out there.

When you start on your journey to better physical fitness (getting lean and having a healthy body fat percentage), you must accept the fact that there are no short-cuts. Your body, young or old, will always react to your diet and exercise routines with hormones, metabolism, lean muscle tissue and/or body fat tissue. Your body has built-in responses', and these have developed as we have evolved from away back when humans were hunter gatherers, not from visits to the local supermarket casually walking up and down the food aisles picking out low-nutrient calorie-dense high-sugar processed foods, etc.

There are loads of fad diets offering the promise of quick results — sometimes, almost unbelievably quick results. Some with little effort and not much time, others by severely restricting your calorific intake or swapping a meal for a shake (yuk). If it's taken you 20 or 30 years to put on that extra 40 pounds, how could you think it would be possible that you could just lose that extra weight (fat) in 2 or 3 months?

Even as you get older your body will do the same thing as a younger body when encountering any sort of significant change in diet and/or exercise. But when you are over 50, you're probably less active than when you were in your 20s or 30s, but more than likely still eating the same amount. Also, as you age, your body creates less human growth hormone. Men will be producing less testosterone while menopausal women will be producing more oestrogen. If you don't take action, then your body will continue to lose muscle (sarcopenia) and store the excess energy as fat. In other words, your body will be storing energy in different ways compared to when you were younger.

For sure, you can only lose weight if you are in a calorific deficit. Our aim is to increase your metabolism to a rate that allows you to be in a deficit whilst eating an amount of healthy food that leaves you feeling satiated and with enough energy to fulfil your new active lifestyle.

Also, with this form of training we must keep in mind that we are training to maximise your weight loss, not your fitness. The aim is to make your body inefficient at using energy (food) by maximising your metabolism. We're not trying to become super strong or become an endurance athlete, albeit you will get some of the benefits that these types of training can provide.

The Benefits of Progressive Weight Training

There is actually a long list of why you should include strength training in your program.

Not only does strength training **increase your physical work capacity**, but it also improves your ability to perform activities of daily living (ADL's). You will be able to work harder and longer with the proper weight training activities.

It improves bone density. One of the best ways you can reduce bone loss and avoid becoming fragile as you age is to add strength training into your workout plan. When we talk about bone health and falls, we're really talking about 3 factors, these being fall, fragility and force. Resistance training and muscle growth can help treat conditions like osteoporosis and provide extra cushioning when you do fall.

Promotes fat-free body mass with decreasing sarcopenia. The lean muscle mass that we all work so hard for decreases with age. If you don't add strength training to your exercise routine, then any excess energy will be stored as fat.

It Increases the strength of connective tissue, muscles, and tendons. This leads to improved motor performance and decreased injury risk.

It improves your quality of life as you gain body confidence. Strength training will not only make you strong but will also help with managing your weight. It can also help with your ability to stay independent as you age as the added strength allows you to maintain daily activities like lifting groceries or even just getting out of a chair.

Develop Better Looking Posture strengthen the muscles that will hold your posture together.

Build Muscle to Improve your Resistance to Injury by using amino acids to continually create new blood cells, regenerate organs, maintain your skin/nails/hair, etc.

Sleep Better & Feel More Energized Sleep is a must and if you can get around 8 hours a night, you'll be more fat resistant.

Build Muscle to raise your metabolism the higher percentage of lean muscle tissue in your body, the higher your metabolism will be. This makes it easier to keep excess weight off. It also means you can continue to enjoy normal satiating amounts of food and avoid those restrictive diets

Note: If you're someone who hasn't exercised for a while or may have some under lying health conditions. Then before embarking on a resistive weight training program it would be advisable to get a health check to make sure that your heart can withstand the demands that working out will bring.

It would also be important for someone to assess if you have muscular or bone issues that may need some work before commencing.

CHAPTER 1

So where do we start?

Well first of all, we need to understand why it's so easy to put weight on, particularly as we age. You know that common saying **'middle age spread'**.

To a certain degree middle age spread does exist, but not because your metabolism slows down, but because as you age, particularly beyond the age of 30, your body naturally starts to lose muscle, usually between 1-2% per year. **Sarcopenia** is the medical term for muscle loss this way, which is very common amongst both male and females from the age of 30 onwards, affecting around about 90% of adults. So, by the time you are 50, an inactive person could have 40% less muscle. It's that loss of muscle that results in a lower metabolism. Note I said lower metabolism, not slower. That's because no matter what age you are your muscles use energy at pretty much the same rate as they always have and it's this fact that we are going to use to help you get your weight back under control.

Loss of muscle is also the main reason why people can become frail as they get older. Our aim will be to reverse the loss of muscle and fire up your testosterone levels and get your body functioning like you were 20 years younger! Before we start delving into workouts or nutrition, we need to understand how things work and what effects they have on our body.

But don't worry, this is a short book and we'll get to the knitty gritty of training very soon.

Let's firstly look at the difference between lean mass and fat mass:

CHAPTER 2

Lean mass Vs Fat mass

Lean body mass equals body weight minus body fat. LBM + BF = BW. (Lean body mass plus body fat equals body weight). The percentage of total body mass that is lean is usually not quoted – it would typically be 60–90%. Instead, the body fat percentage, which is th opposite of this, is computed, and is typically 10–40%.

When people talk about gaining muscle by eating more protein or muscle building workouts, what they're really talking about is gaining or building their Skeletal Muscle Mass. This is because of the three major muscle types – cardiac, smooth (your organs), and skeletal – skeletal muscle mass is the only type of muscle that you can actively grow and develop through proper exercise and nutrition.

Muscle burns more calories than fat. To achieve sustainable weight loss, it is therefore beneficial for one to gain some muscle mass whilst losing fat. Additionally, you might have heard that muscle weighs more than fat. This is a common misconception. Whilst a kilo of muscle weighs exactly the same as a kilo of fat, the difference is that muscle is actually *denser* than fat, which means it doesn't take up as much space as the fat does in your body. That's why if you're working out more, building muscle, you may look slimmer and more fit but still weigh the same amount.

As an example, let's take a 70kg non active person as our example with a current base metabolic rate (BMR) of 1,515 calories.

Their current body weight composition is made up of:

Lean mass = 52.5kg of which approx. 25kg is muscle.

Fat mass = 17.5kg (so currently 25% of their total body weight is fat)

They then train and lose 4kg of Fat and build on 2kg of Muscle (they now have a healthier 20% body fat). This would result in their new weight being 68kg and a new BMR of around 1,715 calories a day (because they now have more muscle) and that's you weighing less and burning 200 calories more per day before you take exercise of any description. That figure varies from person to person depending on body type or DNA and these numbers are only used as an example, but the principle is the same for everyone. So now you can see how increasing your muscle mass is beneficial in achieving a higher metabolism and therefore sustainable weight loss. More muscle = higher metabolism.

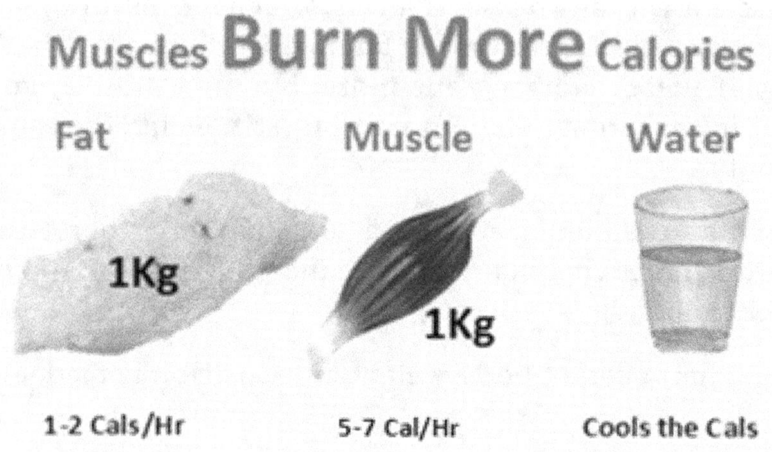

Now let's look at what happens when you exercise those muscles.

If 1kg of muscle burns 5-7 cals/hr at rest and most people can burn up to 15-21cals/hr under exertion and fat only burns 1-2 cals/hr, no matter what (you can't exert fat), then for every extra 1kg of muscle you build on, you could burn around an extra 10-14cals/hr with exercise (less for less intense exercise and vice versa). So previously you may have been burning say 450 cals /hr when doing intense exercise, now with an additional 1kg of muscle you could be burning 468. Let's say you do 10hrs of intense exercise every week, that equates to an extra 180 cals burned per week (that's for each additional 1kg of muscle). And remember every time you move your body, that additional 1kg of muscle will burn more calories. And now your body doesn't have to carry around as much dead weight (Fat), even though you've got more muscle to do so (so you feel more energetic and less stressed). It's just **win win win!**

BMR (base metabolic rate) is the number of calories

you need to keep your body functioning at rest. These basal functions include circulation, breathing, cell production, nutrient processing, protein synthesis etc. But don't take into account how active you are or how much lean tissue you have.

It is also known as your metabolism. Therefore, any increase in lean weight (muscle) or activity will increase your metabolism.

You can use an online calculator like the one found here to find out what your BMR is: Calculate Your Basal Metabolic Rate to Lose Weight (verywellfit.com).

So, the more muscle we have the greater our metabolism will be. So, we want to build muscle.

Now it's possible some of you may be thinking that you will start to look like a professional body builder after this.

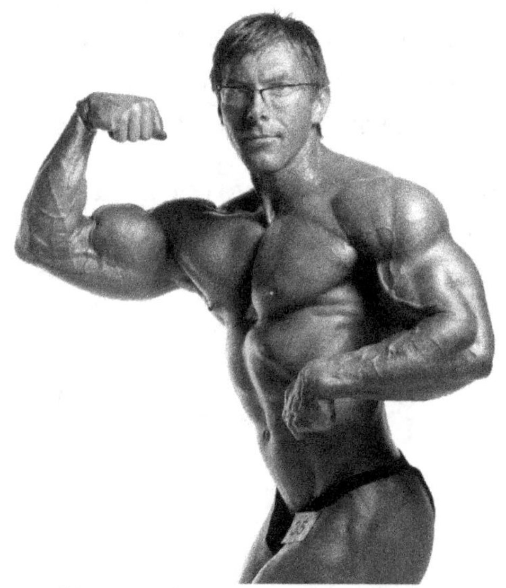

I hate to disappoint, but you almost certainly won't. Not without being genetically gifted, using anabolic supplements along with long periods of intense training. That said, your physical body composition will change and you will look more athletic.

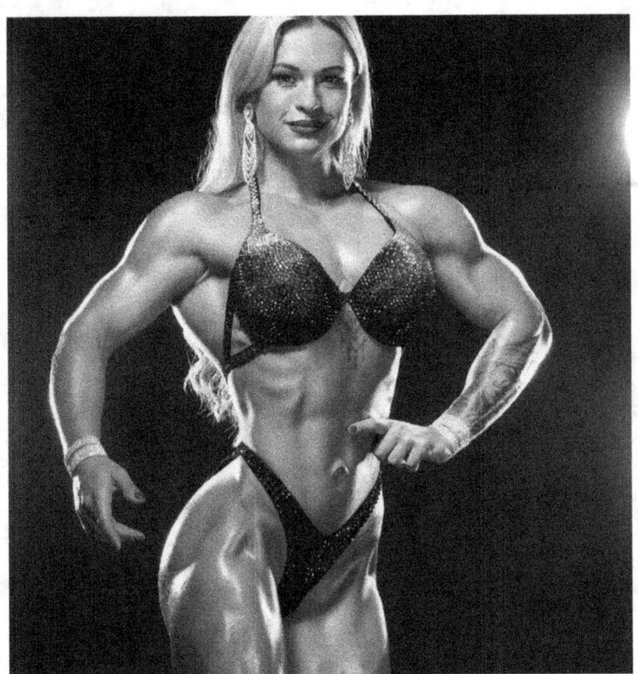

And also, from my experience many females are afraid to lift weights because they fear looking masculine and getting too bulky (like the lady above). There's nothing wrong with looking like that. That woman is strong and that's a good thing. Women who achieve a physique like this put in many hours of training and will be supplementing with artificial testosterone.

Many women, if they do lift, will lift super light weights and perform high repetitions, under the belief that high reps' equates' to muscle tone, not muscle size. This is another common misconception.

The previous image, is what many females think progressive weight training will make them look like . . .

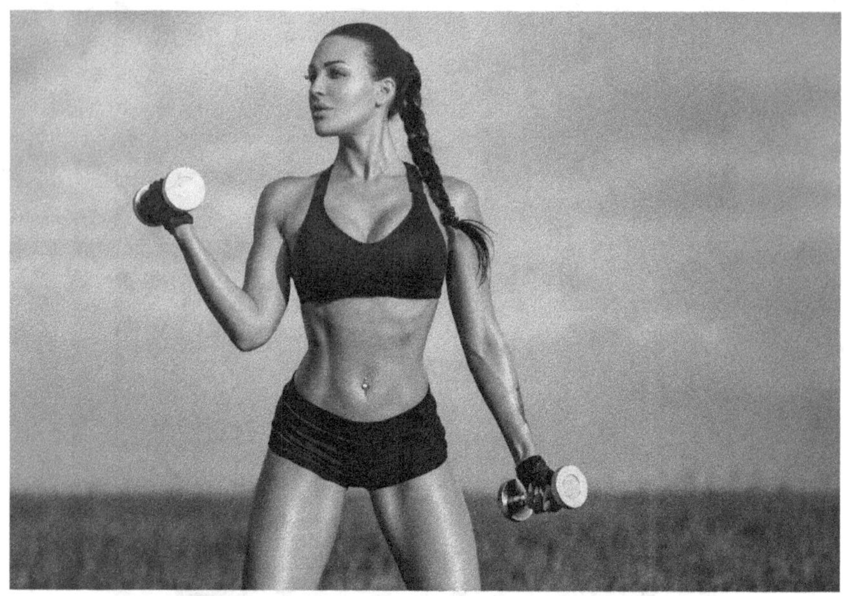

This is what progressive weight training will more likely achieve.

Images like the previous one put females off weight training and understandably so, that is unless you understand more.

Most women can't get bulky even if they wanted to. They simply don't have enough natural testosterone in their bodies to allow them to do so. Women have on average less than a fifth of the testosterone levels of men. As you can see, that's a pretty big difference and means it's harder, if not near impossible for women to bulk up like men.

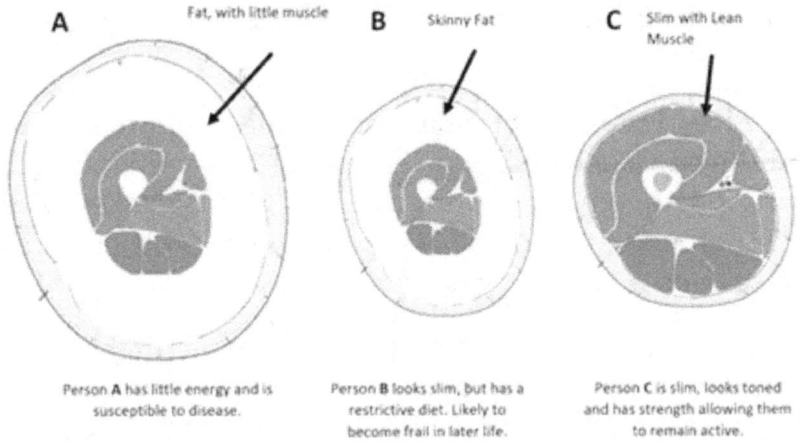

Person **A** has little energy and is susceptible to disease.

Person **B** looks slim, but has a restrictive diet. Likely to become frail in later life.

Person **C** is slim, looks toned and has strength allowing them to remain active.

Image (C) is what progressive resistance training will allow you to achieve. *A growing body of research shows doing weight-bearing exercise can help prevent bone loss (or potentially even build bone), and in turn, reduce your risk of osteoporosis and possible fractures down the line [2].*

A common misconception with females and weight training is . . . you lift weights, you get big and look masculine! But what can we achieve? There's a wide spectrum for you to choose where you want your body composition to sit. It's not just **a)** big muscles or **z)** be skinny, there's many places in between.

It is very difficult to grow even a small amount of muscle mass, let alone a lot. For the average off the street male or female getting big is just not going to happen (unless they resort to steroids, which I don't recommend). Except for the gifted few, most of us are just genetically limited to how much muscle we can build.

For most people currently not participating in any form of strength training, if they striped away their fat, they would be surprised how little muscle they actually have.

Also, there are a number of misunderstandings about building muscle which may lead people to avoid strength training altogether and instead focus on insane levels of cardio along with calorie restricted diets. This can also lead to people becoming skinny fat.

If you are worried that building muscle might make you look bulky instead of skinny, don't! As we have already mentioned, muscle is much denser than fat, meaning that if you weighed the same as you do now, but you had more muscle than fat, you would actually look thinner. Except in this thinner / leaner body, you would be much healthier.

And many women find doing weights in the gym can be quite intimidating, as the weights room is usually full of testosterone fuelled men lifting heavy weights. That can make you feel like your efforts will be watched and judged, when in reality everybody is just getting on with their own workout. The only person judging you will be yourself. So if this sounds a bit like you, then don't worry, everybody has to start somewhere.

And another thing, too much cardio can make you lose fat and muscle (we'll discuss more about that later). **Muscle is your friend** and will help you cultivate the desired hourglass shape that so many women want or the athletic V shape back or broad chest that men want.

When we lose muscle mass, we decrease our life expectancy. The good news is that there are several things we can do to both halt this or reverse the negative effects – and this can be done at any age.

I know that in this book I keep referring to growing muscle and this can create the image of someone getting bigger, when, with weight loss we are looking to reduce our overall body size. We need to start thinking that bigger muscles mean greater potential to burn calories and therefore reduce our body fat. The end result being a leaner thinner body with a higher metabolism which assists us in maintaining our ideal weight and body composition (like the previous female image). We are not training to look like a body builder. For most inactive people if you stripped away all their fat (not really possible) they would look so skinny you would think they were ill.

CHAPTER 3

How to increase your lean body mass

Pump up the protein. Muscle needs fuel—fuel in the form of protein. In an effort to lose weight, it's common to cut back too far on the protein muscles need to tone up. Generally, research shows that women and men trying to increase lean body mass should eat between 0.55 to 1 gram of protein per pound of lean body weight daily.

Most sports nutritionists agree with the research that shows the advised amount of protein required on a daily basis to maintain or gain muscle is usually between 0.55 – 1.0 gram per 1lb of body weight or 1.1 – 2.2 grams per kilogram for active people [1]. There are other studies that show eating less can achieve results, but I believe, as long as you are in the above range you should be fine. At these levels, there is really is no need to take protein supplements. Obviously a very overweight person will get away with a lower amount than a slightly overweight person using this method of calculation as less of their total weight is lean tissue. If you calculate your requirements on lean body weight plus 15% that is about ideal (you can use images freely available on the internet to estimate where your current fat percentage is). Older people need a bit more than younger people, because as you age muscle synthesis becomes less efficient. Also, as you near the level of muscle you want or can genetically achieve you can lower your protein intake to a maintenance level, rather than growth level.

Unlike carbs and fat, there is no need to cycle protein to match your activities, in fact your protein intake should remain consistent, even on non-training days, because your body will need that protein to continue the muscle synthesis process.

Even though a relatively high protein intake is healthy and safe, eating massive amounts of protein long term is unnatural and may cause harm. Traditional populations got most of their calories from fat or carbs, not protein. It's not recommended to go above 4 grams per kilo for sustained periods as this may lead to adverse medical conditions.

It's also recognised that there is a direct relationship between eating excessive amounts of red meat and diseases like cancer, so these types of meat should be taken sparingly. Everything in moderation.

An easy way to judge you are getting the right amount of protein in each meal is to visualise your protein portion as being the same size as the palm of your hand.

Here are 12 terrific sources of lean protein:

1. Fish
2. Seafood
3. Skinless, white-meat poultry (chicken turkey)

4. Lean beef (including tenderloin, sirloin)
5. Skimmed or low-fat milk
6. Skimmed or low-fat (Greek Style) yogurt
7. Nuts
8. Eggs
9. Lean pork (tenderloin)
10. Beans
11. Chickpeas
12. Lentils

Progressive Resistance Training is a strength training method in which the overload is constantly increased to facilitate adaptation (muscle growth). Progressive resistance is essential for building muscle, losing weight, and getting stronger. Progressive Resistance Training initiates the process of Hypertrophy.

In most cases, what people consider to be strength training or resistance training really isn't. If you want to offset muscle loss due to aging, then you have to be training at quite a significant overload level. No less than 60% of your max and working up towards 70-85%. You can't recruit your muscles if you aren't working them hard enough. If you go to the gym 3 or 4 times a week and only lift 5kg dumbbells, then you won't achieve anything, there will be no stress and therefore no progression.

Our body adapts to exercise and needs to be constantly challenged in order to continue to see muscle growth and improved levels of fitness. Doing the same thing day after day with moderate weights may maintain the muscle and strength you have already built, but you are unlikely to see improvements or growth. If your goal is to lose weight, it puts you at risk for a weight loss plateau, that frustrating time when your weight loss starts to stall.

I see so many people attending the gym and doing more or less the same workout (and they're working hard) over and over again and they get next to no results (I know, I was one of them). Well, that's because they are not progressing with overloading the muscles. No progression / overload = no change, it really is that simple. There's also little point in going beyond 15 reps with any exercise as you are now just increasing muscle endurance (which, for an endurance athlete might be what they want), but you are not creating myofibrillar hypertrophy.

What is muscular hypertrophy?

There are two types of muscular hypertrophy:

myofibrillar: growth of muscle contraction parts.

sarcoplasmic: increased muscle glycogen storage.

Which type to focus on depends on your fitness goals. Myofibrillar training will help with strength, speed, muscle growth and fat loss. Sarcoplasmic growth helps give your body more sustained energy for endurance athletic events. So, for our goals (weight loss) we'll be concentrating on myofibrillar hypertrophy.

To build muscle through progressive resistance training, you need to have both mechanical damage and metabolic fatigue (when you can't lift another rep at that weight). When you lift a heavy weight, the contractile proteins in the muscles must generate force to overturn the resistance provided by the weight.

In turn, this can result in structural damage to the

muscles. Mechanical damage to muscle proteins stimulates a repair response in the body. The damaged fibres in muscle proteins result in an increase in muscle size (this is known as hypertrophy).

How Muscle Hypertrophy Happens:

When you start exercising a muscle, first there is an increase in the nerve impulses that cause muscle contraction. This on its own can result in strength gains without any noticeable change in muscle size.

As you continue to exercise, there is a complex interaction of nervous system responses that result in an increase in protein synthesis. Over time (usually months), the muscles start to grow larger and stronger. There are two essential components necessary for the growth of muscles—stimulation and repair.

Stimulation

Stimulation occurs during the contraction of the muscle (during the actual exercising). Each time a muscle is exercised, it contracts. This repeated contraction during a workout causes minute damage to the internal muscle fibres. These muscle fibres are broken down throughout the course of a workout. Once damaged, these fibres now need to be repaired.

Repair

Muscle fibre repair occurs after the workout (when you are resting). Your body produces new muscle fibres to replace and repair the damaged ones. You produce mores fibres than there was before the damage, and this is where the actual muscle growth takes place.

Although the process of hypertrophy is pretty much

the same for everyone, the results can be quite different, even in people doing the same workouts. This difference in results can be because of the genetic make-up of each individual person's muscles. Genetics can affect muscle growth in a number of ways:

Degree of growth

Speed of growth

Shape and appearance of muscle

The end results for individuals may depend more on your dedication to your workouts and your body type, rather than the workout plan that you choose. You have to work to the point of metabolic fatigue (muscular failure) to create the largest stimulus for muscle hypertrophy.

CHAPTER 4

What Does My Body Type Mean?

There are three basic human body types: **the ecto-morph, the mesomorph, and the endomorph** [4]. Despite what it might feel like at times, you're not completely bound to one category or the other. Your lifestyle, genetics, history, and training style all play a part in how you look, and you can definitely change it over time.

An **ectomorph** tends to be thin and struggles to gain weight as either body fat or muscle. They can eat piles of food and stay looking the same, even when gaining muscular weight is their biggest goal. Often referred to as hard gainers in the gym world.

The **mesomorph** has a middle-of-the-road build that takes the best of both worlds. They tend to have wide shoulders, a narrow waist, relatively thin joints, and round muscle bellies. About 80% of us fall into this category.

The **endomorph** tends to gain weight and keep it on. Their build is a little wider than an ectomorph or meso-morph, with a thick ribcage, wide hips, and shorter limbs. They may have more muscle than either of the other body types, but they often struggle to gain it without significant amounts of accompanying body fat.

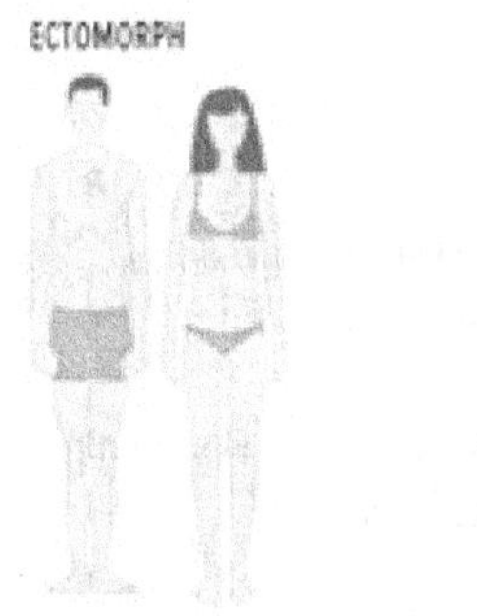

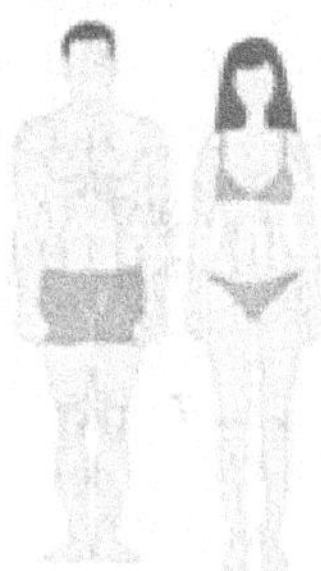

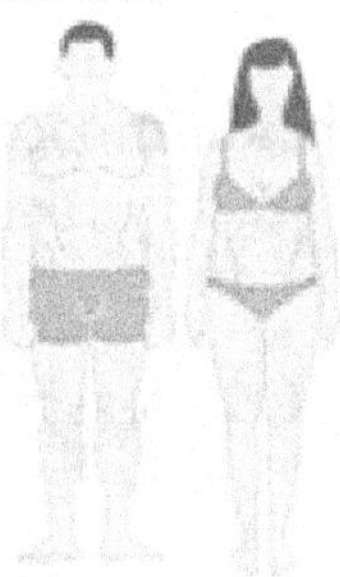

In order for our body to use Hypertrophy to build muscle we need to be in an anabolic state.

Anabolic State: An anabolic state means that your body is building or repairing tissue. When you rest, your body goes into damaged muscle tissue and begins repairing it. It's during **rest**, not exercise that you actually increase your muscle size.

Since anabolism and catabolism are parts of your metabolism, these processes affect your body weight. Remember: When you're in an anabolic state, you're building and maintaining your muscle mass. When you're in a catabolic state, you're breaking down or losing overall mass, that can be both fat and muscle (loss of muscle is atrophy). Anabolism is where your body uses all that protein in your diet as a building block for muscle.

Insufficient protein in your diet, means no anabolic state, no hypertrophy and therefore no change in your body composition.

Muscles don't keep growing (or grow at all) if your

body is not in an anabolic state. Which is why some body builders take anabolic steroids.

Since the point of body anabolism is to build and maintain muscle tissue, there is no way to be in an anabolic state without first stressing your muscles. The best way to induce stress in them is by exercise.

Progressive Resistance Training is one of the most effective ways to progressively stress the muscles.

Therefor to have hypertrophy you need to both stress the muscles and provide them with the right nutrients from your diet.

There are many ways to achieve progressive resistance, and hence hypertrophy:

Increase the weight you're lifting. Do the same number of reps and sets each week, but increase the weight you are using. You should only increase the weights by 2 percent to 10 percent of your current RM (1 x Rep Max) load at a time. The RM load is the maximum amount of weight you can lift one time. For example, if you can lift 50 pounds once, you should only increase the weight you lift with each rep by 1 to 5 pounds each week. You don't want to overdo the increase in the load, as this may lead to injury.

Increase the number of reps. Use the same weight for each workout but increase the reps each week. Not usually beyond 15. When you go beyond 15 reps, you are generally only increasing your muscle endurance (sarcoplasmic hypertrophy} which won't create myofibrillar hypertrophy.

Decrease the number of reps. Intermediate to advanced trainers can lift heavier weights for fewer reps, known as heavy loading. When doing heavy loading, you increased the rest time between sets to two to three minutes.

Increase the number of sets. A typical weight training workout for people with the goal to lose weight will involve about two to four sets of each exercise. If you're a beginner, one set may be enough to build strength and endurance but, as you get stronger, you'll want to eventually work your way up to two to four sets, resting about 30 seconds to 90 seconds between sets, depending on how heavy you're lifting.

Shorten the rest between the sets. If you're doing straight sets, e.g., three sets of squats or three sets of push ups, you'll typically have a rest of about 30 seconds to 90 seconds between sets. One way to challenge your body and increase intensity is to shorten the rest between sets. If your form starts to suffer, drop the weight a little. You can do compound sets, where you do 2 exercises for the same muscle group one after the other (no rest).

Lengthen the time under tension. This is how long your muscle fibres are under stress. Use the same weight and reps but slow down the exercise. For example, one count to lift the weight, three counts to lower the weight.

Time Under Tension (TUT) is essential for muscle development. You should always be trying to ensure your muscles stay under tension when preforming an exercise for hypertrophy. One method of doing this is to keep the muscle you are working 'squeezed' never relaxing it, particularly on the eccentric part of the movement (the lowering part or stretching part). Squeezing a muscle throughout the exercise helps keep it under tension.

To be able to achieve this, you need to learn the exercise movement first. Only then can you start using this squeeze to create a strong 'mind-muscle connection' to the muscles you are working. If you don't do this, then you'll struggle to engage the muscle fully. This is obviously easier to achieve on isolation exercises than it is on compound exercises where multiple muscles are involved.

You also have to place enough load through the muscle, or it won't grow. That said, it doesn't mean that the weight needs to be super heavy. Once you have perfected the exercise technique (good form) and have good mind-muscle connection, you can start to load the muscle. When you do load the muscle, it shouldn't compromise your form or that squeeze, if it does, the load was too heavy. Remember, **good form trumps everything**

The optimal time under tension for muscle growth is between 30 and 90 seconds per set, so any weight that doesn't lead to failure by the end of your last set in about 90 seconds really wasn't heavy enough or held under tension long enough. That can be acceptable for your first set or two where you are warming the muscles and building up the weight (load), but not for your last set.

If you can perform an exercise for over 90 seconds before reaching failure, you're not likely to achieve myofibrillar hypertrophy (muscle growth). You only improve your muscle endurance (which for endurance athletes, that may be what they are trying to achieve). This also applies to quite a few of the popular but misguided exercises like press ups, chin ups, curls etc. where you see people pumping out high reps.

Any exercise that is light enough to be done for high reps will, because you turned it into an aerobic exercise have no impact on your muscle development and is pretty much a waste of your precious gym time if weight loss is your goal.

By utilising and varying your resistance training we can continue to progress without using very heavy weights which may lead to injury. However, to achieve results, we **must always** be trying to achieve resistance progression (overload), at least until you reach your end goal (desired weight loss).

One last thing, **leave your Ego at home!** Don't try to lift heavy weights to impress others in the gym, it just leads to bad form or worse, injury.

Good form trumps everything!

CHAPTER 5

Managing your Macronutrients

Macronutrients are the nutrients we need in larger quantities to provide us with energy: in other words, Fat, Protein and Carbohydrate.

Total calorie intake is important; however, it's just one piece of the puzzle, Macronutrients are the main contributors of calories in our diets and each has its own unique effect on the body. We therefore need to manage our macros to match what we are trying to achieve.

For building muscle, we need to increase our protein and good fats (good fats are used to help you convert protein to muscle). On days where you will be doing aerobic exercise (say cycling, running or walking etc.), then you would want to fuel your glycogen stores to maintain your endurance, so on these days you need to increase your carbohydrate intake whilst controlling your other macros.

There's been a lot of advice out there recently that is advising you to cut out carbs, but carbs are not inherently bad, they actually provide the energy you need to stay active. However, eating too many high glycaemic carbohydrate calories can lead to weight gain because your body will store any extra energy as fat. So, while you won't need to forgo carbs, you'll want to practice portion control with carb-heavy foods to avoid exceeding your carbohydrate requirements. Your carb intake should match your activity levels. That is, eat more carbs when your being active and less on rest days.

Eating too many carbs might also negatively impact your blood sugar levels [6]. Normally, blood sugar serves as a source of energy for your cells; your tissues can take up the sugar in your bloodstream and convert it into usable energy (glycogen) to fuel your active lifestyle. But refined carbs — sugar or "white" carbs like white bread and pasta — digest quickly and can cause a pronounced spike in your blood sugar levels. Your body responds by releasing hormones (insulin) to lower your blood sugar levels but often ends up overcompensating and causing a blood sugar "crash" that leaves you feeling tired and hungry.

Over time, eating too many carbs can negatively affect your ability to control your blood sugar levels. People who eat a higher glycaemic index diet, i.e., one full of carb-rich foods that cause blood sugar spikes, face a higher risk of developing type-2 diabetes (did you know that a person who has diabetes carries the same health risks as someone who has already had one heart attack?).

Unlike fats and carbs, there's no real reason to ever withhold your protein intake. You won't get more fat loss from eating less protein. Protein is very satiating (about 30% of protein calories are used just digesting it. It's

5-10% for carbs and 3-11% for fats), most people will actually get less fat loss when avoiding protein. So even when your primary goal is fat loss, don't skimp on protein on any day.

Whether your program is full body workouts or split routines, you'll still need to consume the recommended amounts of protein every day. Even if you slightly exceed the recommended amounts, there's no real drawback, other than perhaps cost. And if that additional protein results in you eating less fats and carbs, that can result in more fat loss over time.

As you can see, all three macronutrients have important roles in the body. But the ratio in which you consume them can affect various health outcomes, such as muscle gains, endurance, appetite levels, and heart health, diabetes etc.

So, we can see that you can't just exercise and not eat healthily, and you can't just eat healthily and not exercise. Eating protein rich foods is key to building muscle, but so is doing effective resistance exercises if we want to build muscle.

So basically, to build muscle we just need a well-balanced diet that matches our activities and / or strenuous exercise?

Not quite, there is another quite significant factor and that's hormones. As we age, we naturally reduce our production of growth hormone (GH) and testosterone (to a lesser extent women as well). These hormones are key to muscle building.

But, not to worry, progressive resistance training also

induces your body to start producing these hormones. Ok, so you're not going to be 17 again, but you will notice the difference in your energy levels and the changes that it makes to your body composition.

As a note, there is no real reason for anyone to take protein supplements, you should be able to get enough protein from the food in your diet. Plus, eating is way more satiating than drinking a protein shake.

If you do feel that you want to take a protein supplement for the reason of convenience. I.e you don't need to prepare a meal. Then be very careful and check the nutritional values on the label, because some of these products have very high amounts of sugar and you have to ask yourself are you really going to be training hard enough and long enough to use that carbohydrate energy intake. Because if you don't, then your body will store the excess energy as fat and that's exactly what we're trying to avoid. Remember **manage your macros**.

CHAPTER 6

Boosting Your Growth Hormone

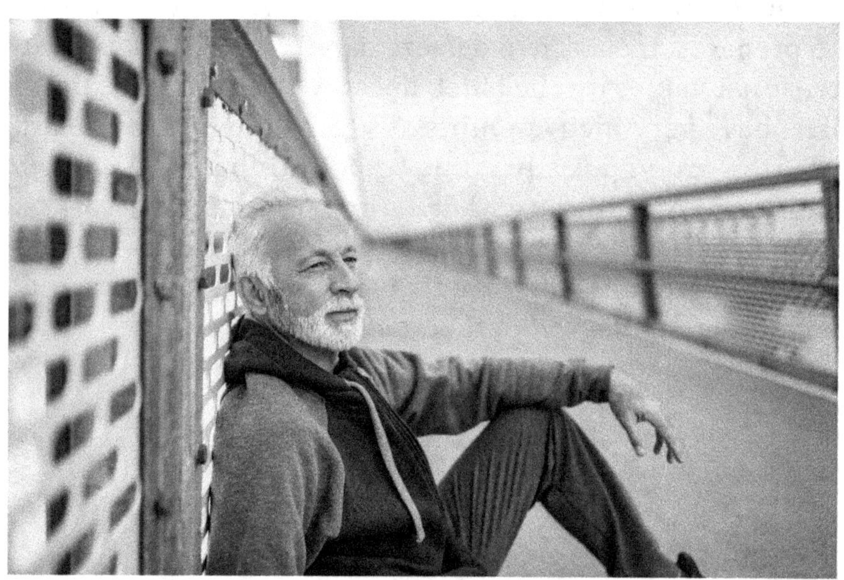

Hormones are the other factor that play a huge part in overall quality of life, as well as gaining muscle & losing body fat. It's the difference that either makes you feel unstoppable and high after a workout, or low on energy and unable to progress effectively whilst training.

Optimal hormone levels are key in order to progress with weight loss. All it takes is a few different habits to get your body working for you, not against you. Studies have shown that there is no definite evidence that artificial GH treatments work. You are far better of increasing your GH through diet, exercise, and sleep.

7 ways for to boost growth hormone and

lose body fat

Proper meal planning, placing protein as a priority. Protein rich foods are not only satisfying, but they promote weight loss and the potential to build muscle mass. It also lowers insulin, whilst helping to improve blood sugar levels. These kinds of foods help to promote hormone balance due to their nutrient value. Try to source only lean meats and seafood for their richness.

Get plenty of sleep when you can. Cortisol is released when we lack sleep. The by-product of this is increased hunger hormones and a decrease in androgens. Because glycaemic control is also lowered, your body will not be able to handle as many carbs. If you can allow for that little bit of extra sleep by going to bed earlier, or having a short nap during the day, you will greatly increase your levels of growth hormone.

High Intensity Interval Training (HIIT). Anaerobic training produces the release of many positive hormones, keeping your metabolism active and giving you a positive state of mind. It's a primary component of the release of growth hormone for an improved body composition, improving oestrogen metabolism and testosterone. Using weight training and sprints as a weight loss and muscle building strategy, also allows you to improve your insulin receptors, allowing for more carbohydrates to be enjoyed and utilised properly by the body (instead of being stored as fat).

Make vegetables of high importance – avoid refined carbohydrates.
Hormones are affected by refined carbs and sugar. It causes blood sugar spikes, reducing insulin sensitivity over time, and leads to a huge release of cortisol. Vegetables (plant sources) on the other hand are a very healthy carb alternative, filled with fibre (keeping you full as well as being quite low in calories) lowering inflammation whilst improving hormone balance.

Don't be afraid of adding fats to your diet. Fats provide the building blocks for our bodies to manufacture hormones. It's also used to make the outside lipid layer of cells. Healthy Fats such as avocado, and omega 3 rich salmon, improves cellular singling, making them more receptive to insulin. This then results in optimal hormone balance and health.

Manage your stress levels. Cortisol is a key hormone that increases the potential of your body to store fat and decreases muscle growth in the process. Learning how to manage stress is a key part of the weight-loss process – as well as building muscle mass. Try to meditate or take a walk in the park. Try to find what works for you when it comes to lowering your stress levels' and getting you back to baseline.

Progressive Resistance Training: Weights too have a great effect on hormones, helping your body to shift from fat storage to fat burning. It will move your body towards using fat for energy, thereby eliminating fat all over your body, as well as enhancing the shape of your muscles. A lot of people mistake cardio as the only way to lose weight. Too much cardio can decrease your muscle mass even further, and then set your basal metabolic rate even lower. I'll explain this in more detail later. You want to increase your baseline metabolic rate by increasing your muscle mass, losing fat via proper nutrition and weight training.

CHAPTER 7

How Long Does It Take to Build Muscle?

This is a common question that people ask when they start exercising. However, it all comes down to where you are starting from. Because the reality is:

We all have to start somewhere.

A former athlete or gym goer will have an easier time building muscles and losing fat than someone who is inactive and overweight. There are mainly two reasons for this:

The pre-selected genetic blueprint of the athlete.

Work ethic of an athlete.

While countless variables play a role in influencing your success in the gym, it can all be traced back to those crucial factors. And this saying still holds merit:

"Hard work beats talent, when talent doesn't work hard." Tim Notke basketball coach – Team USA [3].

People with average skills, average genetics and average work ethic. As long as they keep improving on their craft, they will still succeed.

Not immediately – but over time they will.

That said, the more muscle that you have when starting an exercise programme, the greater the changes you will see during training.

Here's what results you can expect if your main goal is building muscle. **Warning:** Genuine muscle growth without performance enhancing drugs like anabolic steroids takes considerable time.

Of course, these time periods can vary individually depending on your body type, genetics and work-ethic. You might see results sooner, or maybe even later than the average person.

The first month of progressive weight training is likely to yield little gain in muscle mass. It's not a matter of how hard you workout or how much protein you eat. Your muscles have to go through the initial stage of adjusting themselves to the process of breaking down and building up.

I should say here that this is the period where you are likely to suffer from delayed onset muscle soreness (DOMS). That's the pain and stiffness you feel in your muscles several hours to days after unaccustomed or strenuous exercise. The soreness is felt most strongly 24 to 72 hours after the exercise. It is thought to be caused by eccentric (lengthening) exercise, which causes small-scale damage (microtrauma) to the muscle fibres. It's usually worse after exercises where higher reps have been done.

Having said that, you are likely to see some reassuring changes in your body. Your muscles will begin to tone up and blood flow will increase, making them look slightly larger and more defined.

You'll also see some increases in your strength. 15% - 20% gains after 6 weeks is not unusual.

Once you are past the initial DOMS stage, then the muscle building process begins, with every exercise progression leading to an increase in the muscles exercised.

Just to give you an idea of what may be possible, but it will vary from person to person, with some doing better and others worse depending on genetics and body type. After the initial period and assuming that you consistently follow the correct training regime and no supplements are taken, a male may initially expect to add around 0.2 - 0.4kgs of muscle per month and a female 0.15 – 0.25kgs per month. It takes a long time to build muscle. This is different to a body builder who may be going through a bulking period. We're trying to increase muscle whilst avoiding any increase in fat.

I recommend training 3-4 times per week (continuously!).

For quicker results, consider training with an experienced gym goer or hire a personal trainer to boost your progress tremendously.

More information on this can be found at www.life-hack.com [5]

Month 1 – 3

Eat (Fuel) – Sleep (Rest) – Exercise (Gym) – Repeat.

Your motivation is at your peak at this point. You will tell your friends and family about your new workout regime. You will notice slight differences in your appearance, which are very slight if any.

You will experience strength gains on your training because your body finally realises that you have muscles you can use.

After about 6 weeks, if you were to look at your muscle cells under a microscope, you would see that the slow and fast twitch muscle fibres are getting bigger. This means you are adding more protein into your muscles, and you will start to see your metabolic rate increasing so that even when you are asleep you are burning more energy."

You're now over the sore bit. You won't be getting so fatigued or feeling tired and if you're working out properly, your muscles shouldn't be stiff or sore.

Month 3-6

This is the stage where most people fail. You will be going to the gym consistently, yet the visual results can't be seen yet. It's the big dip in the whole process. It is working, it's just that you are most likely to still have a layer of fat hiding your results.

Your goal in this phase is to build a habit around your gym visits. You are unlikely to still have the all-in mentality that you had in the first 3 months. You will seek sustainability. Breaking news! It will still be hard work.

But in the end, it's all worth it. You must believe in the routine and remaining consistent will get you the results you want.

Month 6-12

This is the time where the average person starts to see considerable results from their training.

Your muscles will be visibly bigger and noticeably more efficient, meaning you'll enjoy better endurance. You'll be fitter, so you'll be able to work at a higher intensity, lift heavier weights and run, row, or cycle at a higher intensity, which can increase the feel-good endorphins filtering into your brain.

People will start to see a difference in your body shape, as you now have a lower body fat percentage and more defined muscle. As a frequent gym-goer you'll start to have a good feeling every time you go. It's an exciting time as you can now see the rewards coming from your

hard efforts.

Month 12- 24

After 12 months, your bone health will have significantly improved. You see people who were osteoporotic return to normal bone health, and that's massive in terms of reducing your risk of fracture or becoming frail.

While you might think frequent training will only change your body shape, your character will be impacted too.

Your friends and family around you will notice. You're more confident, assertive and happier with your self-image. You feel confident and sure in your abilities because you have achieved what you set out to do. You'll be more active because you now enjoy activity.

But perhaps the best thing that will happen after

maintaining your exercise regime for a year is the fact that going to the gym is now an ingrained habit.

A point worth noting, as you progress with your training, you may find yourself tempted to train harder for longer or participate in another active sport or pastime. Avoid the temptation to do another high intensity activity on the same day as your gym workout, particularly at the outset as you will not leave enough time for your body to recover. Remember you build muscle when you are resting, not exercising. The exercise creates the stimulation for muscle synthesis, the rest period allows it to repair and build.

If you do too much exercise, you will put yourself into a catabolic state. This is where your body burns muscle as well as fat and carbs for energy. You will also start to crave high glycaemic foods which can result in fat gain. Any loss of muscle will result in lowering your metabolism, which is the opposite of what you are trying to achieve. Add extra calories to that from the food cravings and you will see your weight and body fat composition heading in the wrong direction.

If you want to keep active, just go for a walk. Walking is low intensity and keeps you in the fat burning zone. An hours' walking requires little to no recovery and won't hold back your body's ability to build muscle.

To begin with, less is more.

CHAPTER 8

Split Training

Because muscle growth takes place when our body is resting, it's important that we allow enough time for this to happen. A good way to achieve this is to split your workouts so that some muscle groups are resting whilst others are being worked. The most effective splits are segmenting upper and lower body. When splitting your training by body parts, you have a more effective chance at hitting a higher volume of training, as you allow your muscles to rest from a section of the body (say your upper body) then the next day, hitting the lower body. Resistance training is generally low intensity which keeps you in the fat burning zone.

HIIT (High Intensity Training being the exception)

It looks a little like this example:

Split one: Shoulders, Back and Abs

Split two: Hamstrings, Quads, Glutes and Core

Split Three: Biceps, Triceps and Chest

I prefer to allocate 2 days on and one or two days

off to allow the body a full recovery and increase muscle protein synthesis (hypertrophy). I would also couple the training week with a higher caloric consumption day – which just means you consume more food than you normally would (preferably more protein). This is great for igniting your metabolism and replenishing muscles.

Final word on split training

If you want your muscles to grow, they need to be trained frequently. Genetics does have some inherent bonus factors when it comes to building muscle mass, but your true ability to gain muscles mass is determined by how quickly you recover, so you can get back into the gym and smash it. It is very important you split your training into lower and upper body sessions. So, when you are hitting the lower body on day one, then on day two your lower body rests, whilst we workout the upper section.

As we progress with the progressive resistance training and you start to see the results, it's likely that you will want to start more advanced workouts targeting specific parts of your body to achieve better muscle balance or performance for a sport or pastime you participate in, like say cycling or running etc.

For this we use Isolation exercises. Some of which I have listed towards the back of this book.

CHAPTER 9

Consistency

I can say with some certainty, that success comes from consistency of training. Keeping the motivation to train, despite your initial enthusiasm can be one of the hardest things to maintain. However, there are some simple and practical ways that you can adapt into your life, that will help maintain your motivation.

Plan your exercise routine. A great way to maintain motivation is to plan your routine. What are your fitness goals, is it weight loss or body composition? What do you have to do to achieve them? What's going to make you get out there and train. I find that goal setting in my gym diary usually helps me. Having a plan to lift a certain amount of weight or certain number of reps or lose a certain amount of weight in a short period, gets my motivation going. I'm constantly setting mini targets for individual exercises.

Have different options. Always make it easy on yourself by planning different routines. What I mean by this is, find an alternative to every little barrier that appears in your way. Don't want to go outside because the weather is bad, then hit the gym. The piece of equipment you want to use in your gym is taken. Then have an alternative exercise planned that uses a different piece of kit as a backup in your training program. If you don't want to leave the house, because you're not in the mood or another activity or work is in the way. Then how about a little session with resistance bands or dumbbells in your own home instead. I have eliminated excuses by buying some dumbbells, and resistance bands. They all help towards my goals, and when I feel like training at home, I use my equipment. It's easy, and I am still able to get a workout.

Convenience is key. If a gym is too far away from your home, or somewhat inconvenient for you, you'll come up with every excuse to stop you going. The best alternative is always to pick a gym that's either close to your home or work. Find a way that will work best for your lifestyle. Remember, if it's enjoyable you will do it. If it's convenient, you will be more likely to go. If you can combine these two attributes, then the motivation to train will be there.

Read more about training. Especially about people similar to yourself who have achieved their goals. This can be the spark to set your motivation alight again.

Could you have time off? This probably seems the opposite of what you want to do, but time away can help to motivate you. Don't get too stressed, because there will be times in your life when you can't train - and that's ok. Constantly pressurising yourself to keep going will leave you feeling exhausted and stressed (and you now know what effects stress has on fat loss). Your decision to exercise or not is neither right nor wrong - it's just your decision. Give yourself a chance to experience exercise as an opportunity to feel good, but not an obligation that you have to go to the gym.

Set your alarm clock. The alarm clock isn't just for a morning wake up call, so how about setting an alarm call before your workout? If you like to work out at a particular time, allow yourself a good few minutes before you need to get ready. This can be your reminder that it's time to get your gym kit ready.

Sign up to a personal trainer. You will be committed to turn up to your paid for session. Your trainer will set your routine and push you to achieve the results required for you to progress. Some gyms have basic weight training classes', and these can be useful when starting out.

Get a training partner. You can get good results by just having a regular training partner who is trying to achieve similar results to yourself. You'll turn up just because you don't want to let them down. There might even be a little friendly competition between the two of you.

Look back at that gym diary you've been keeping and see how far you've come. Reflect on what you've achieved so far. Don't let the effort you've put into achieving the results you've made so far go to waste.

Discipline. This is a crucial one for those times when you're not motivated. Have the discipline to make sure you do that workout.

I know how hard it can be to stay motivated, but I find some things work better than others. Music can be a key motivator for some or reading up on health and nutrition, but this will vary from person to person. Having said that, if you feel like resting or just working out from home, then feel free to do that. A few days away isn't going to harm your results, it may. even give you more motivation to work harder through your next workouts

CHAPTER 10

Is cardio a good way to burn fat?

Depending on what kind of cardio you are doing, for sure it can help you with fat loss, there is no doubt about that. The only thing that can cause actual fat gain is when the energy we consume is greater than the energy we use. Cardio does result in some energy to leave the body – which can create a deficit (weight loss).

However, you may have some situations in which doing cardio can cause the likely hood of gaining weight, or not losing weight at all. What you need to understand is that cardio is not the only reason for this.

Below I will highlight some points about cardio, which will help you to understand its effects on the body, and what benefits or downfalls it may have to achieving fat and weight loss over time.

With time, your body adapts to cardiovascular exercise, making it less effective. You may have experienced this from your past training, as you get fitter, you need to up the distance, train harder and faster – or else there is no way to keep up the same metabolic benefits. The amount of exercise you would have to do, leads to diminishing returns, increasing the likelihood of muscle being burned as fuel and cortisol being produced due to increased stress on your body. You end up chasing cardio, as you never seem to get enough to get the results you want.

More cardio leads to increased hunger and inevitable food consumption. You just can't resist it, long bouts of cardio makes you a lot hungrier than normal, and many people unfortunately end up eating more. There are also many misconceptions about having to fuel yourself with carbs before, during and after your workout, which may in fact lead to a larger consumption of high glycaemic foods. This can halt or inhibit your ability to create a calorific deficit, making your efforts pretty much a waste of time as far as weight loss is concerned. If you are doing some kind of light exercise, you most likely will not need to fuel up as much as someone cycling 50K etc. This is just something to consider, because our chosen nutrition (managing our macros) plays a big part in inhibiting and increasing your caloric burn potential.

Elevated cortisol, due to stress and increased activity to match, can make it harder to lose body fat. High cortisol levels encourage your body to store fat, can make you resistant to insulin and can cause inflammation. This, therefore, stops our bodies ability to burn fat for energy. Cortisol induces cravings of those high carb, refined sugary treats. This is a hormone imbalance, and more likely to occur in people who are plagued by chronic stress. Stress leads to growth hormone and testosterone suppression. This factor leads to fat gain, especially in the belly and mid rift area.

When you couple high cortisol with cardio, you are more likely to gain fat. Just doing excessive cardio alone can raise your cortisol levels. If you have to get up to the level of constantly increasing your duration and intensity because the body is not responding, you can bet that fat gain will be inevitable down the track. This is why as a long-term strategy; cardio is not the best option to choose.

Long Cardio Sessions, can lead to injury and aging. Hard-core aerobic activity creates a significant demand on your body. Whether you are running, swimming, or biking—continuous aerobic stress brings on degeneration and ageing. The ageing occurs because initially your body will use glucose (in the form of glycogen) for energy and later will start consuming healthy body tissue like collagen and muscle for fuel. The average person only has about 90 minutes' worth of glycogen stores in their body (endurance athletes can train to become more efficient at using their glycogen). Once your glycogen is used up, your body starts consuming your healthy body tissue which can prevent exercise induced growth. If your muscle tissue wears down, so does your stored glutamine and the production of growth hormone, thus, as muscle is reduced, the skin has less firmness and sags more. Its why long-distance runners can end up looking like POWs.

Cardio coupled with a restrictive diet. This can lead to people becoming skinny fat. What's skinny fat? Skinny fat is when people might look healthy on the outside, but on the inside, their bodies may be at high risk for a number of health problems. The term "skinny fat" is actually a popular term that describes a very real medical condition called sarcopenic obesity. This condition refers to an individual who may have what would be considered a normal/healthy weight, but metabolically, this person shares many health characteristics as someone who is overweight or obese. They are likely to become frail in later life which can lead to injuries and loss of mobility.

There are of course some very positive benefits from doing cardiovascular exercises. Cardio is great for your heart health and regular cardio can help reduce your bloop pressure, reduce your bad cholesterol and increase your good cholesterol. Some form of cardio should always form part of your exercise regime. I would recommend 2 - 3hrs of light cardio per week, like walking or 30 – 90mins of more intense (vigorous) cardio like running or cycling. Just don't do high intensity activities on the same day as your resistance workouts. Also, if you work too hard on your cardio sessions in the earlier stages of your fitness, you will raise your heart rate beyond what you can efficiently work at and quickly put yourself into a catabolic state (remember this is when you're breaking down and losing overall mass, both fat and muscle). You should try to keep your heart rate within 45% of your spare heart rate capacity. Your spare heart rate capacity is the difference between your resting heart rate and your maximum heart rate.

Example: Someone with a resting heart rate of 55 and a maximum heart rate of 175 would have a spare heart rate capacity of 120 beats (175-55). So for low to moderate intensity cardio (fat burning) they should keep their herat rate below 45% of their spare capacity 120 x 0.45 = 54 + 55 (resting rate) = 109 beats per minute.

As you get fitter, your spare heart rate capacity will increase as your resting rate will decrease and your maximum will increase. Although affected by age (capacity decreases as we age), the more capacity you have, generally the fitter you are.

Lots of intense cardio makes you feel tired and crave high glycaemic foods (you know that time after a big day out when you raid every cupboard in the kitchen looking for food). This is probably the biggest reason why beginners quit in the early stages of joining to the gym. The real benefits of going to the gym come from progressive resistance training, not cardio.

The chart below is another way to calculate if you are working within your fat burning range

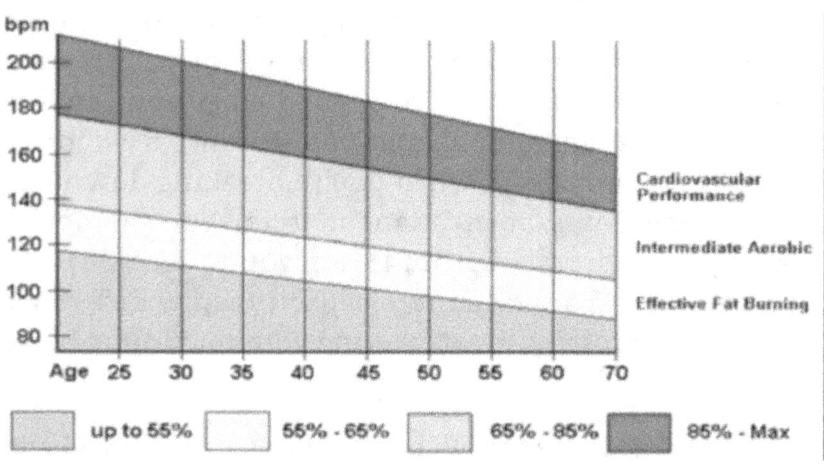

I see numerous beginners turn up at the gym and they go hammer and tongs on the treadmill or cross trainers, sweating profusely. They're working way beyond their current sustainable fitness level and then several weeks later they find they can't sustain the effort, they're too tired due to muscle loss as well as fat loss, so stop going to the gym and are never to be seen again.

Concentrate in keeping your cardio sessions at a pace where you can keep your heart rate within your fat burning zone. Low to Moderate intensity (at least on the days of your gym workouts).

So hopefully now that we understand the process of building muscle a little better and the benefits that has on your metabolism, we can now start to think about what type of workouts you should be doing.

Like I said earlier, I prefer to split my workouts into segments for upper and lower body. As you become more advanced and want to target specific areas, then you may consider splitting your workouts even further by doing isolation exercises for specific muscle groups.

Once we start our exercises, we must always be mindful of not overworking ourselves and allowing plenty of time for rest and recovery. Remember it's the recovery period were your body repairs and builds muscle. Too much exercise can lead to muscle loss and therefore a reduction in your metabolism. Which again is the opposite of what we are trying to achieve.

For that reason, I recommend a gym workout to be no longer than 60 mins. But you must work for the whole of that 60 minutes. If it takes you longer than 60 mins you are either working too hard, resting too much between sets or talking too much. You would be surprised how many people use the gym to socialise and then forget what they are actually there for.

LOG IT OR LOSE IT!

Get a Gym Diary. It's a must.

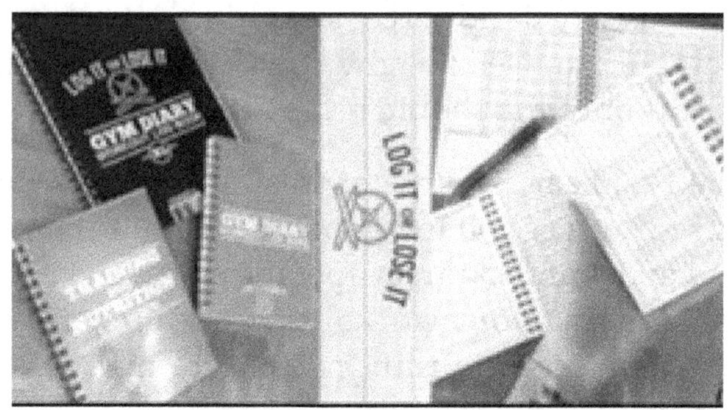

In order to track your success, it's also important that you record all the details of each workout. Only by knowing where you started, can you easily see what gains you are achieving.

It also allows you to see what adjustments you need to make to each exercise in order to ensure that you continue to progress. Remember it is progressive resistance training. If you don't progress, you won't see the results that you are trying to achieve.

When people don't see the results they are looking for, it's almost always as a result of not following the overload (progression) principle.

The next diagram is an example of what a completed gym diary for one exercise might look like. There is no set rule, as long as it works for you, but keep it simple.

Here you can see an example of progression on the bench press. You can also put little ticks against a set if it was easily manageable, meaning there's the possibility for you to increase the resistance the next time you do that exercise providing your form was good. A little cross means it was at your limit or you lost form. So, you would stick at that weight / TUT (time under tension) or even drop the weight until you can achieve that weight with good form.

Remember, **Good form trumps everything!**

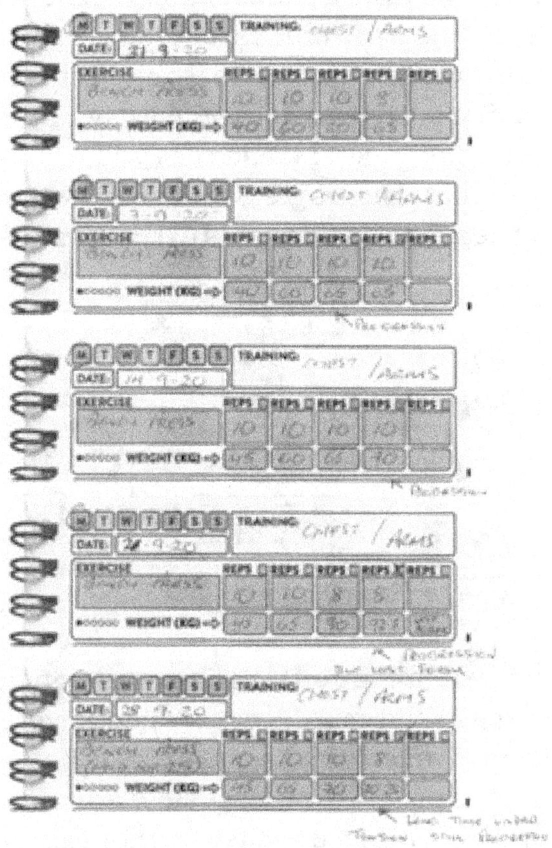

It won't always be as linear as shown here. There will be some days where you don't see some progression or you may even see a dip, for various reasons, perhaps you're just tired, or feeling a little under the weather. And that's ok, just so long as the general trend sees you progressing. You may also find that you progress quicker in some areas than you do in others, and again that is natural and ok.

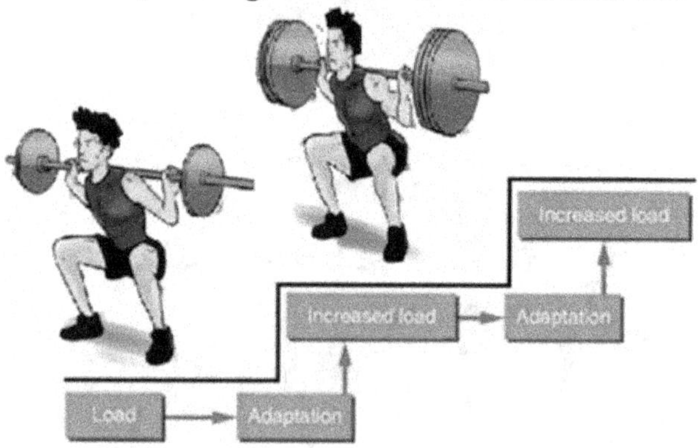

In the beginning you will likely see some significant gains in strength and muscle endurance as your body discovers you have muscles you can actually use. As you progress, the rate of progression does slow down. This again is quite natural as explained earlier, it's not easy to build significant amounts of muscle in a short time. You have to be in it for the long term. Only then will you see the sustainable results.

However, there is an end game. Once you reach your goal, whether that be your ideal weight or physical composition, then the process becomes a little easier (it doesn't stop) but you can tailor your workouts to maintain your results, rather than look for further change.

CHAPTER 11

A good healthy diet is a must

If we want to have sustainable weight loss, then for sure your diet will have to reflect your weight loss goals. This doesn't mean eating less, but it does mean avoiding junk foods and heavily processed foods. You should eat like your life depends on it, because ultimately it does. You may not have any issues just now, but down the line things could change and by then it might be too late.

You need to learn what healthy food looks like. Most of us are familiar with the advice that we are supposed to eat five helpings of fruit and veg every day for a healthy diet, but what does this actually look like? Are carbohydrates really a no-no? And is all fat bad?

We need to learn to choose low glycaemic plant-based foods for your carbohydrate intake (foods that determine how slowly or quickly they can spike an individual's blood sugar). Some fats are required in your diet for muscle synthesis, you just need to learn to choose healthy fats. Try to choose a variety of different foods from each of the groups to help you get the wide range of nutrients your body needs to stay healthy.

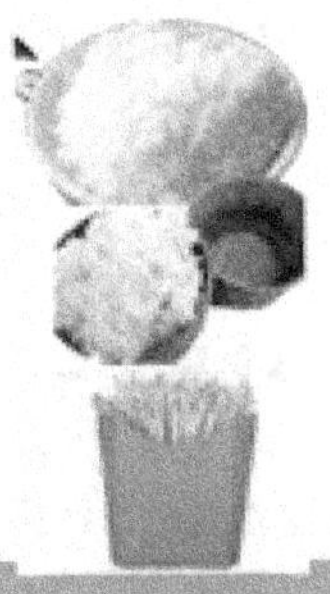
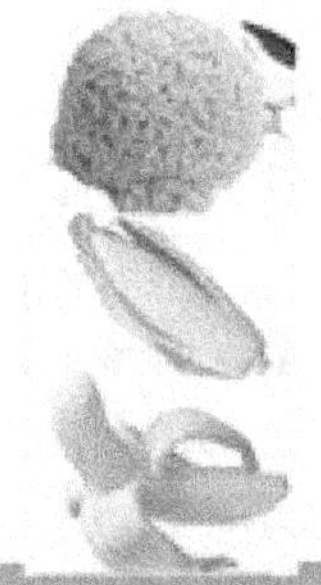
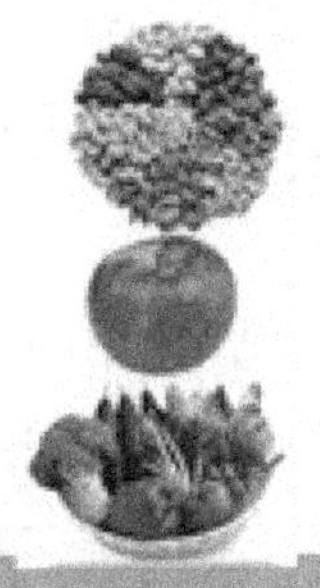

High glycemic		Moderate glycemic		Low glycemic	
Glucose	100	Corn	59	Apples	39
Honey	87	Sucrose	59	Fish Fingers	38
White rice	85	All Bran	51	Butter beans	36
Cereal	80	Brown rice	50	Low fat yogurt	33
Whole meal bread	72	White Pasta	50	Navy beans	31
Potatoes	70	Sweet potatoes	48	Kidney beans	29
White bread	69	Porridge	46	Lentils	28
Shredded wheat	67	Peach	42	Milk (full fat)	27
Mars Bar	65	Whole wheat pasta	42	Fructose	20
Raisins / Sultanas	64	Oranges	42	Soy beans	18
Bananas	62	Blueberries	40	Peanuts	13

And remember to manage your macros to reflect what type of exercise you are taking.

So, does maintaining a good healthy diet mean I can no longer have treats like a takeaway or chocolate or that ice scream on a hot sunny day?

Absolutely not, we all like to have a treat now and again, just not too often. Remember, **you can't out train a bad diet!**

Don't think of yourself as being on a diet, but rather that you have a nutrition program you're working to. You won't be eating less, just better. You should feel satiated. You have to fuel your body for those workouts and your new active lifestyle (that can mean eating more than you were). Overall, having a cheat day once a week is going to help you lose weight, but it shouldn't be done too often, that's more important if you have 25+ pounds to lose. A cheat day will let you look forward to something when sticking to the clean diet gets tough on the other days and will hopefully re-motivate you to stick to your nutrition program for the rest of the week. For me, Friday is my cheat day, couple of beers, some snacks, maybe an occasional take away. It's ok, my metabolism is working so much faster now, it has little to no effect on my overall results.

The stricter you are with your diet, the faster you are likely to see the results, but on the other side that strictness may be less enjoyable or sustainable and therefore may result in you giving up before your target is reached.

Set yourself a nutritional program that you can enjoy and therefore sustain. Remember we're trying to make changes that we can maintain for a lifetime, not just for a quick fix.

There is no quick fix!

CHAPTER 12

Progressive Weight Training Workouts

Progressive weight training, also known as progressive overload, is the gradual increase of stress placed upon the body during training.

The principle here is to continuously increase the demands on the musculoskeletal system so that we can make gains in muscle size, strength, and endurance. In its simplest terms: to increase muscle size and strength, you must progress by lifting more weight, adding more reps or sets or increasing the time under tension. Thus, making your muscles work harder than what they're used to. Without this progression, there will be no improvement.

It sounds simple enough, yet most of us know someone who's been a hard-working gym-goer for years and ends up getting nowhere. In nine out of 10 cases, they didn't follow the overload principle.

In the first week, you want to train at about 60 - 70 percent of your max, moving the weights up in 2-5 percent increments each week, until you reach about 85 percent.

This holds true primarily for compound exercises. Note that the smaller more isolated exercises will progress in smaller steps

After about 4-5 weeks you should be reaching a level where you can train at about 80-85% of your 1 rep max and now your program needs to change to start progressing your max.

Obviously, an absolute beginner won't know what their 1 rep max is, and you might need to spend a couple of workouts with a personal trainer or experienced gym goer to help you identify this.

It is also very important in order to avoid injury, that each exercise is performed with **good form** and again a personal trainer or experienced gym goer should be able to help you with this. You can also search YouTube for videos on how to perform any particular exercise correctly. Remember, **Good form trumps everything!**

Initially for beginners it's best to concentrate on compound exercises with one or two isolation exercises first. **Compound exercises** are multi-joint movements that work several muscles or muscle groups at one time.

CHAPTER 13

Why are Compound Exercises Important?

Why should your early workout routines focus primarily on compound exercises? Isolation moves, after all, target specific muscles, are easier to do, and can generally mean lifting lighter weights. So why not just build your fitness routine around them? There are a few reasons...

1. Compound exercises work more muscle

If each compound exercise is working more muscle, then in a shorter time, you can get a lot more work in by using compound movements (you get more bang for your buck!).

2. Compound exercises are more useful

Muscles rarely work in isolation in the real world. So, training them to work together is a more effective way to build functional strength."

Functional strength exercises build real world everyday strength and often resemble everyday movements. Performing the squat is similar to standing up from a seated position, whereas doing an isolation move like the leg extension is similar to, well, nothing that you would do outside the gym. Both exercises build muscle, but compound exercises are more like real-world activities.

3. Compound exercises burn more calories

Because compound movements engage more muscles (i.e., they are more metabolically active than isolation exercises, they also increase the amount of energy (calories) you burn. As a result, a routine that includes the pull-up, deadlift, farmers walk and squat will ultimately burn more fat than one that includes the chest fly, straight arm row, bicep curl, and leg extension etc.

4. Compound exercises make you stronger

Since compound exercises engage more muscles than isolation exercises, they can be used to move heavier weights. That leads to more muscles being brought under tension, which you now know is a key factor for growth. And the reason is that it creates more micro damage within the muscle, which the body then repairs and builds (hypertrophy), making you stronger.

As you progress in your ability and get nearer to your target weight or body look, then you can start to split your workout and also introduce some isolated exercises which allow you to target specific muscle groups in order to change particular parts of your body composition. E.g., your biceps or legs etc.

In the next chapter I have shown some good compound exercises which can be done both at the gym and/or at home with very little equipment.

Assuming you don't have major injuries or movement restrictions, compound exercises should form the foundation of your strength training workouts. Here are a few that can help you maximise muscle growth for all your muscle groups.

Some of the Best Compound Exercises

1. Dumbbell bench press

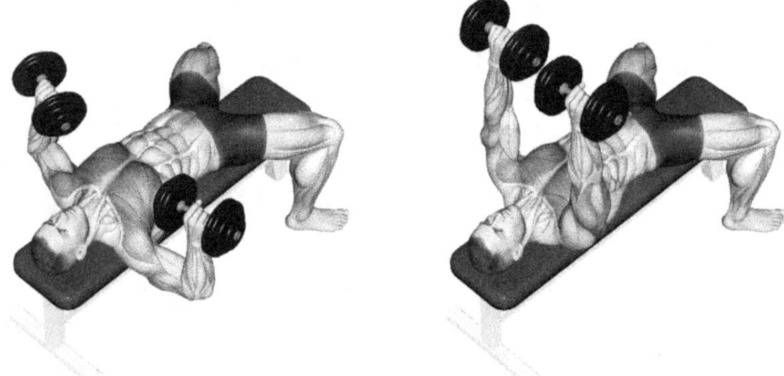

Lie on a flat bench holding a pair of dumbbells directly above your chest with your palms facing forward.

Keeping your feet flat on the floor, your core engaged, and your lower back pressed into the bench, slowly lower the weights to the sides of your chest, keeping your elbows at a 45-degree angle to your body (not flared).

Pause, and then push the weights back up to the starting position

2. The Chin Up

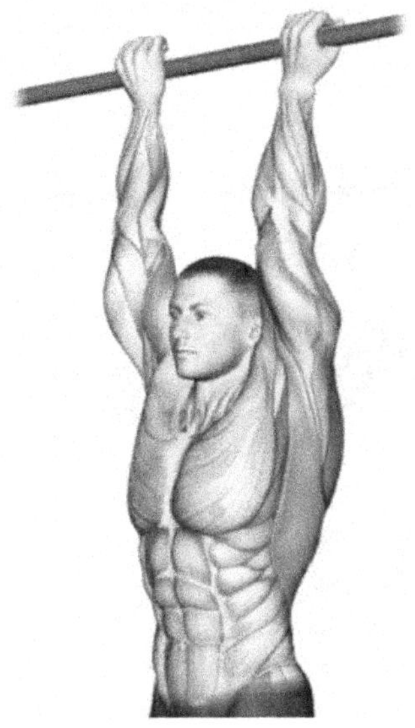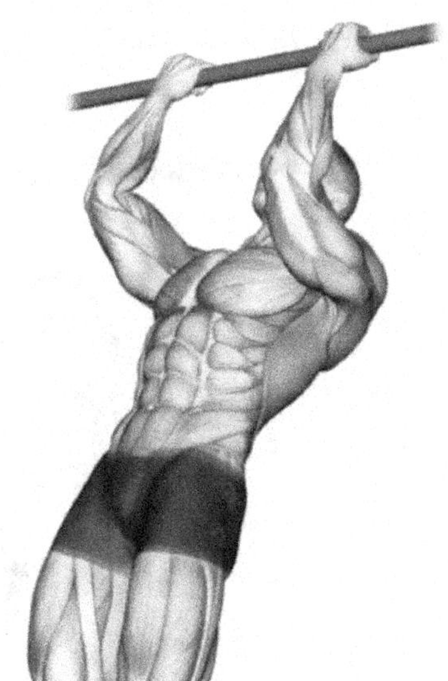

Grab the chin-up bar with an underhand grip that's slightly wider than shoulder-width and hang at arm's length (a position known as a dead hang).

Keeping your back straight and core engaged, pull your elbows to your sides, and squeeze your shoulder blades together to bring your chin above the bar.

Pause, and then slowly lower yourself back the starting position.

3. Dumbbell Dead Lift

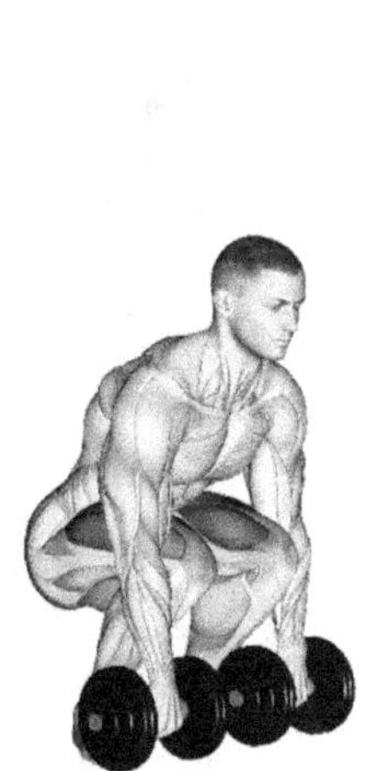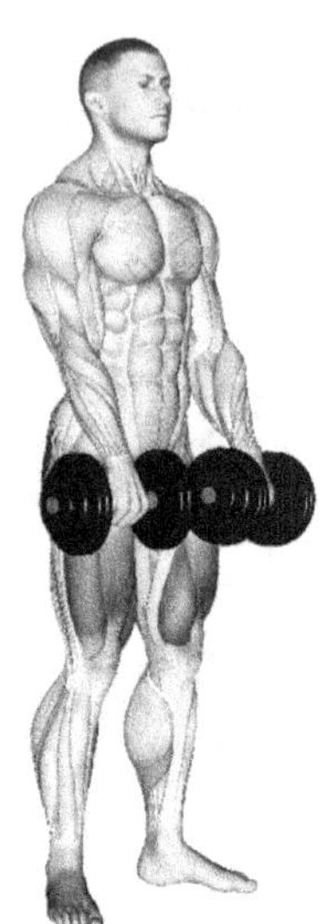

Grab a pair of dumbbells and hold them at arm's length in front of your thighs, palms facing back. This is the starting position.

Keeping your back flat, chest up, and core braced, push your hips back and lower the weights to mid-shin level, keeping them close to your body (your hips should remain higher than your knees).

Pause, and then return to the starting position

4. The Dip

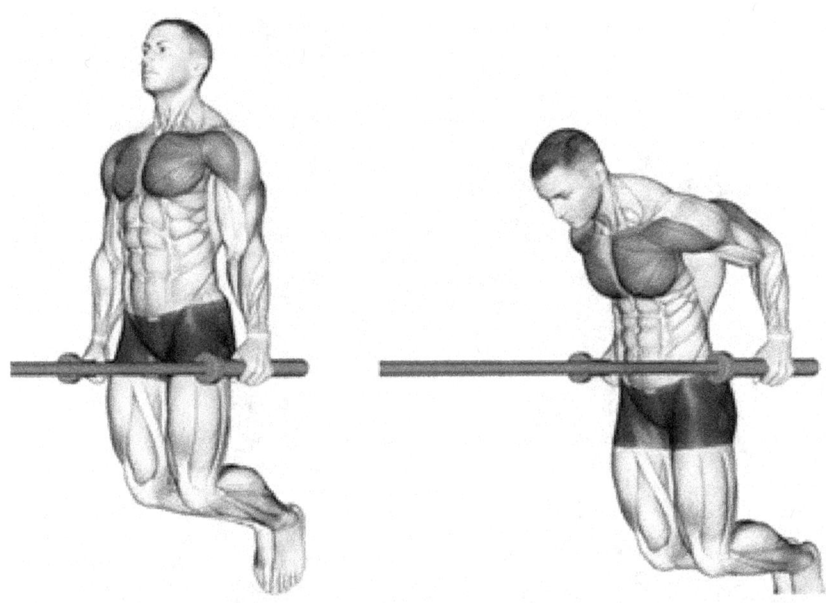

Grab the handles of a dip station and jump or step up to the starting position: arms straight, chest up, back flat, feet off the floor, and ankles crossed behind you. This is the starting position.

Keeping your head neutral and arms close to your sides, bend your elbows until your upper arms are parallel to the floor.

Pause, and then return to the starting position

5. Dumbbell Overhead Press

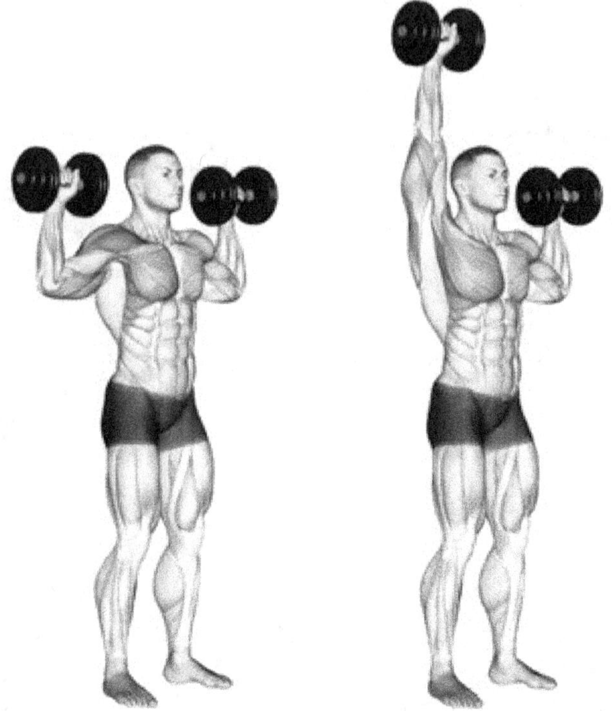

Stand with your feet hip-width apart (step a foot slightly behind you for stability if necessary), holding two dumbbells in front of your shoulders, palms facing each other.

Keeping your back straight and core engaged, press the dumbbells directly over your shoulders until your arms are straight and your biceps are by your ears.

Pause, and then return to the starting position

6. The Farmers Walk

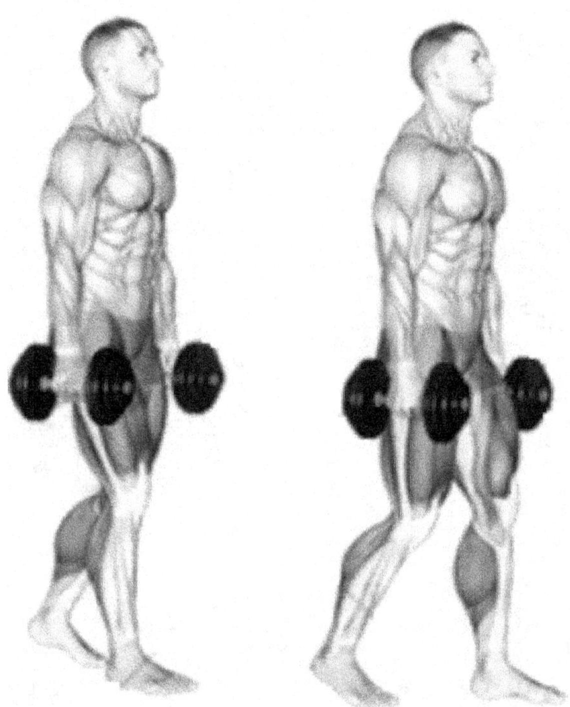

Stand holding two heavy dumbbells by your sides with your palms facing in. Brace your core (as if someone is about to hit you in the stomach) and draw your shoulder blades back and down.

Walk for 20 to 30 seconds to complete one "set."

A good target is to aim to walk with your own body weight for 20 – 25 metres.

7. The Forward Leaning Lunge

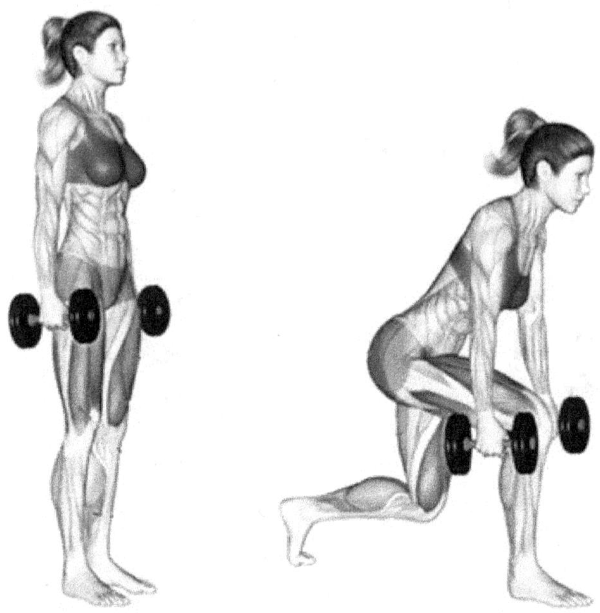

Stand holding a pair of dumbbells at your sides, palms in, with your feet hip-width apart.

Keeping your chest up, gaze forward, back flat, and core engaged, take a large step forward with your right foot and lower your body until your right thigh is parallel to the floor and your left knee is bent 90 degrees. For some people your knee will lightly kiss the ground.

Pause, and then return to the starting position. Repeat, this time stepping forward with the left foot. Continue alternating sides with each rep.

8. The Dumbbell Squat

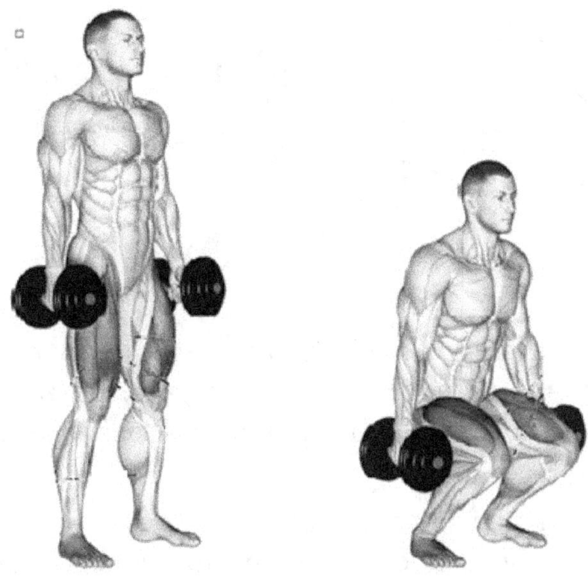

Stand holding a pair of dumbbells at your sides with your palms facing in, your feet shoulder-width apart, and toes pointed forward. This is the starting position.

Keeping your back flat, chest up, and core engaged, push your hips back and bend your knees, lowering your body until your thighs are parallel to the floor.

Pause, and then push yourself back up to the starting position.

9. The Plank

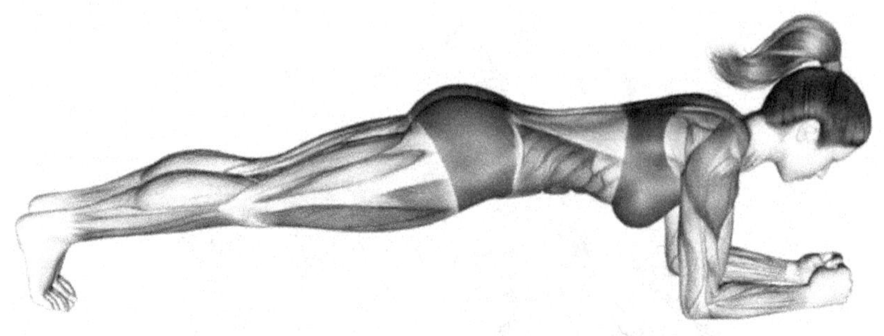

The starting position for this exercise is the same as it is for a push-up – your body in a straight line (like a straight plank of wood) with your hands and feet shoulder-width apart.

Next, squeeze your glutes (buttocks) to stabilize the front half of your body facing the floor and pull in your abs. Be sure your head is in line with your back by looking at the floor about a foot in front of your hands. This takes the pressure off your neck.

Hold this position for 20 seconds when first starting out. As you get more comfortable holding this position, gradually increase the amount of time without compromising your form or breathing. Don't let your buttocks drop as this puts pressure on the lower back and can lead to injury. 4 x 60 seconds is a good target.

10. The Seated Row

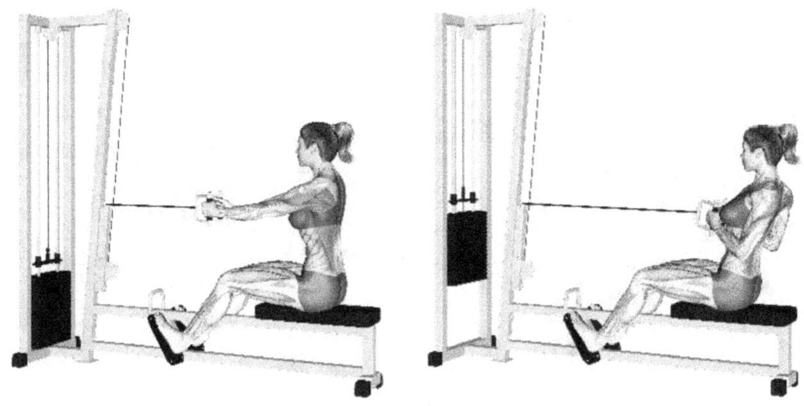

Pull the handle and weight back toward the lower abdomen while trying not to use the momentum of the row too much by moving the torso backward with the arms.

Target the middle to upper back by keeping your back straight and squeezing your shoulder blades together as you row, chest out.

Return the handle forward under tension to full stretch, remembering to keep that back straight even though flexed at the hips. Repeat the exercise for the desired number of repetitions.

11. Ab Roller

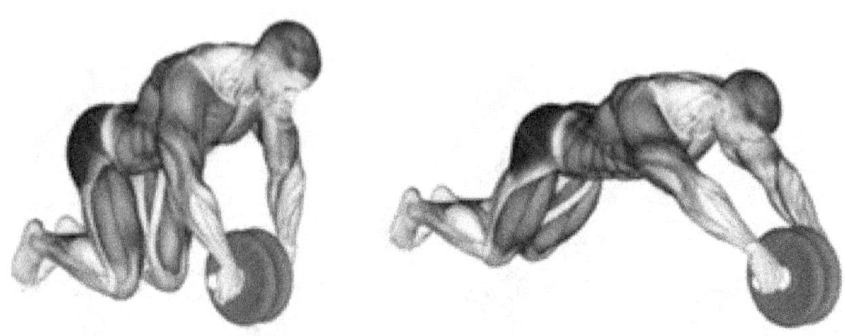

Push the roller out slowly whilst holding the lower abdominals under tension trying not to use the momentum of the roller too much.

Target the lower abs by keeping your back straight and squeezing your abdominal muscles. Hold the out reached position for a count of 1 or 2 before returning to the start position.

Exercises to target specific muscle groups.

Arms (Triceps)

Triceps Dip

Triceps Dumbbell Kick Back

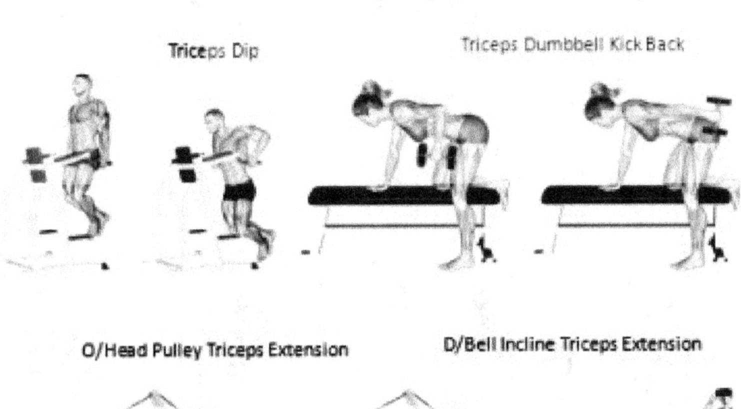

O/Head Pulley Triceps Extension

D/Bell Incline Triceps Extension

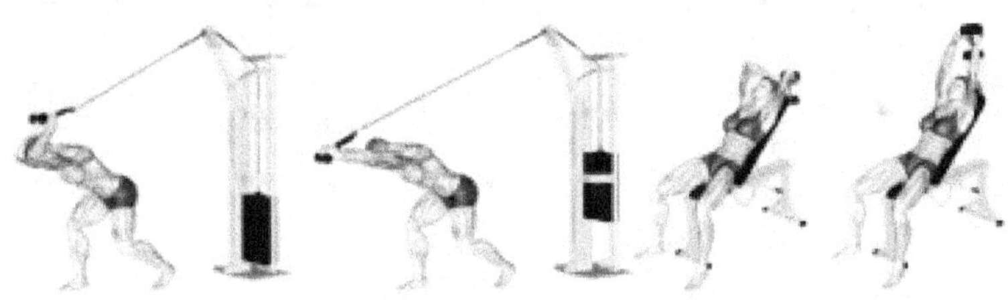

EZ Bar Triceps Extension

Cable Triceps Pushdown

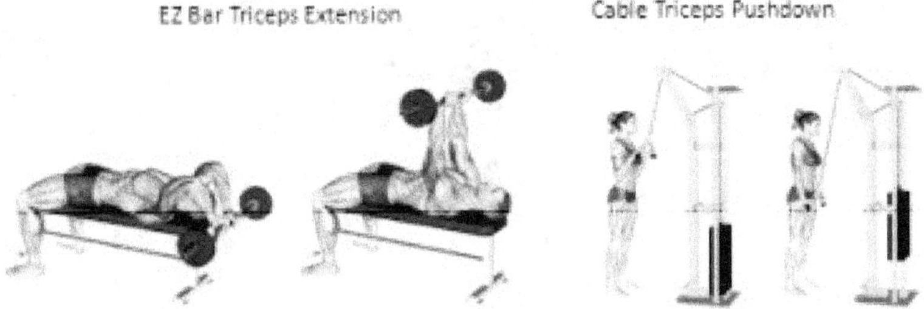

Arms (Biceps)

EZ Bar Curl

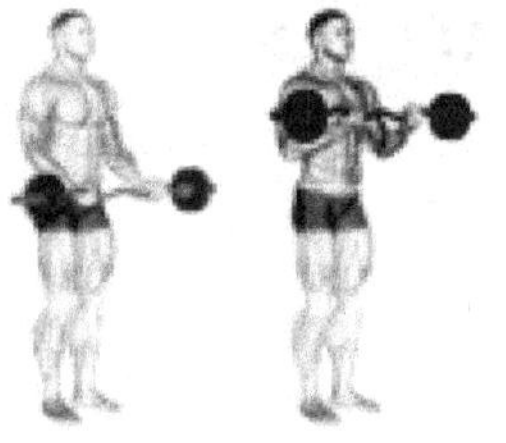

Cable Bar Curl

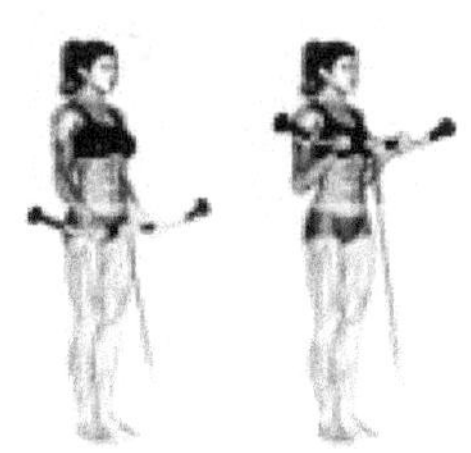

EZ Bar Preacher Curl

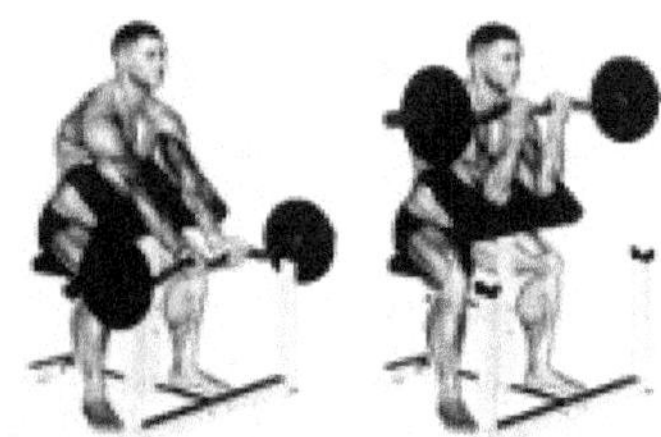

Dumbbell Hammer Curl

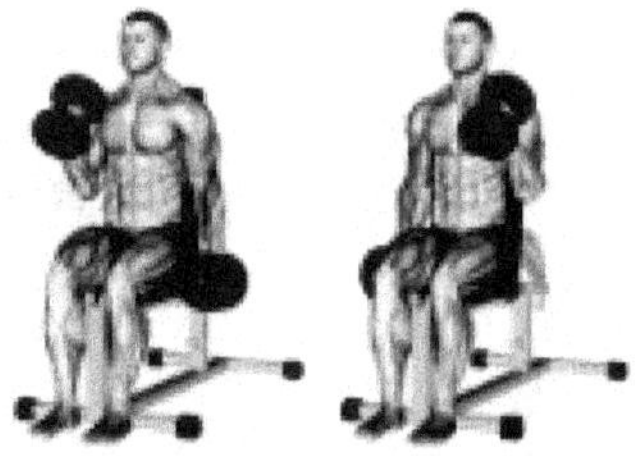

Dumbbell Concentration Curl

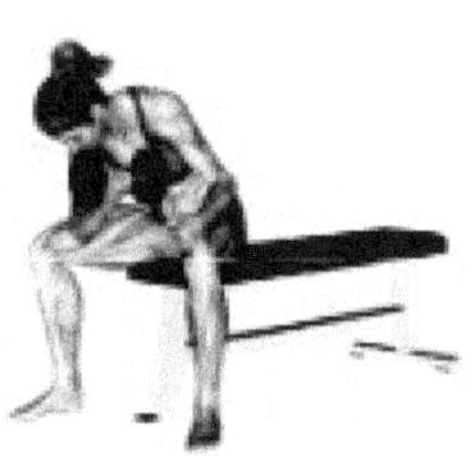

Alternate D/Bell Curl

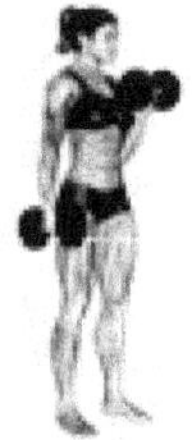
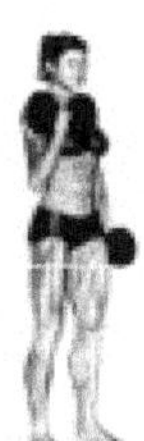

Shoulders

D/Bell Overhead Press

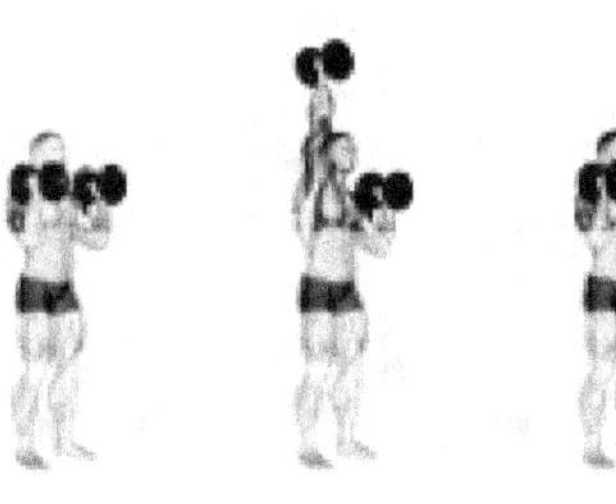

Seated D/Bell Press

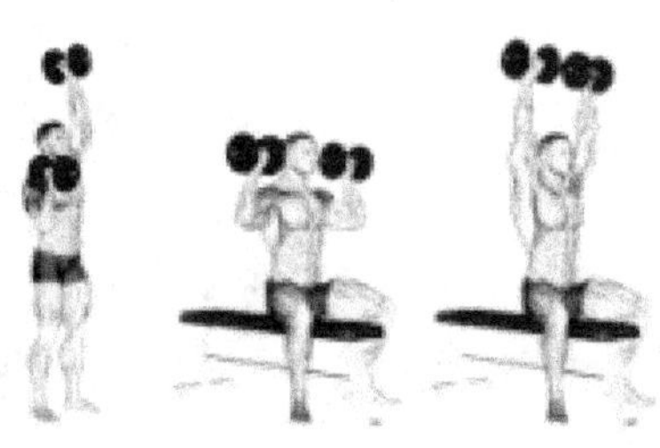

Cable Upright Row

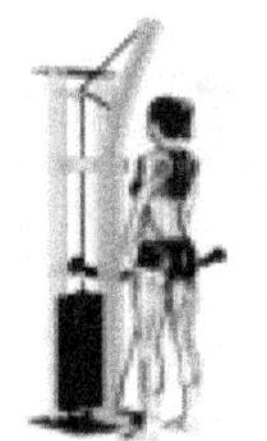

Lever Seated Reverse Fly

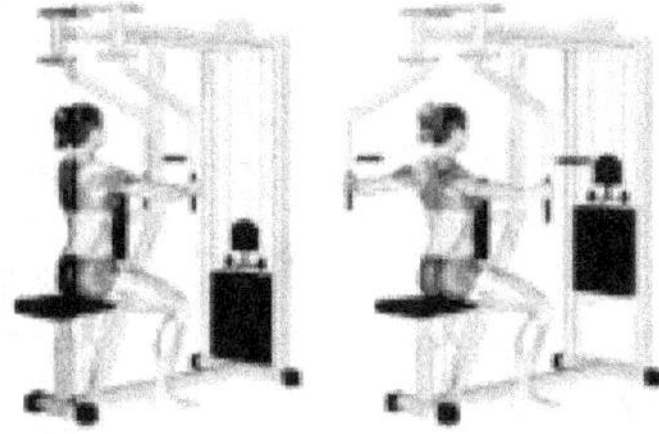

Lever shoulder Press

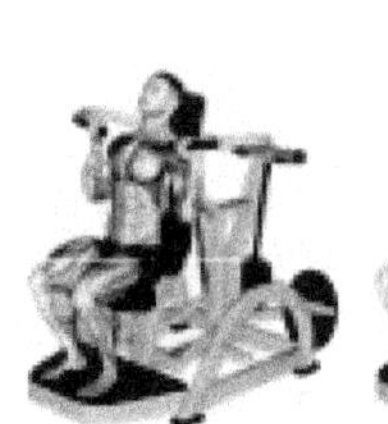
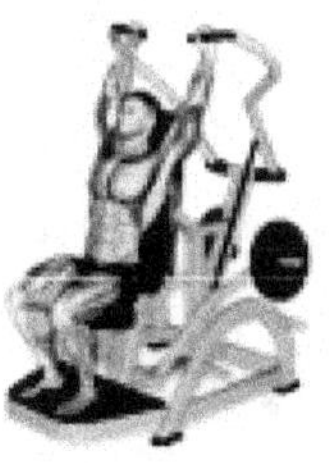

Standing Bent Arm Lateral Raise

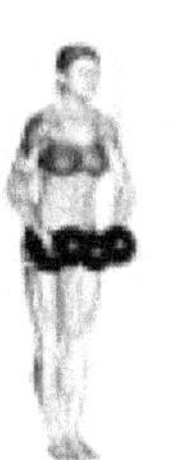
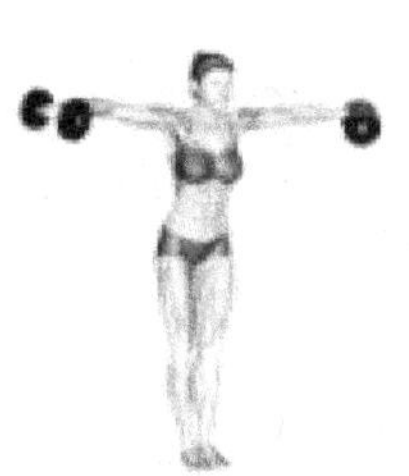

Back

Cable Underhand Pulldown

Cable Seated Row

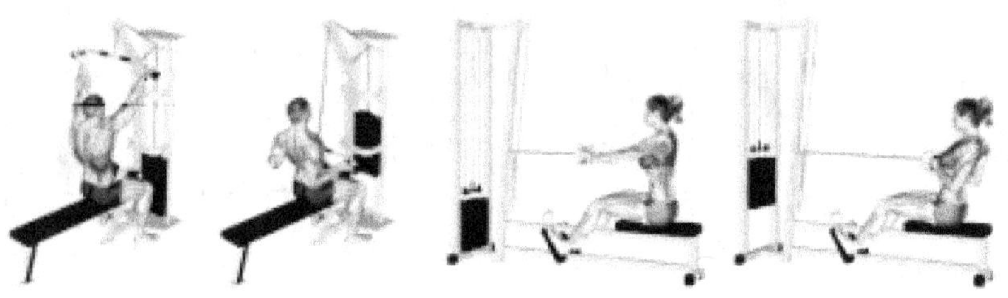

Body Weight Pull Up

Dumbbell Bent Over Row

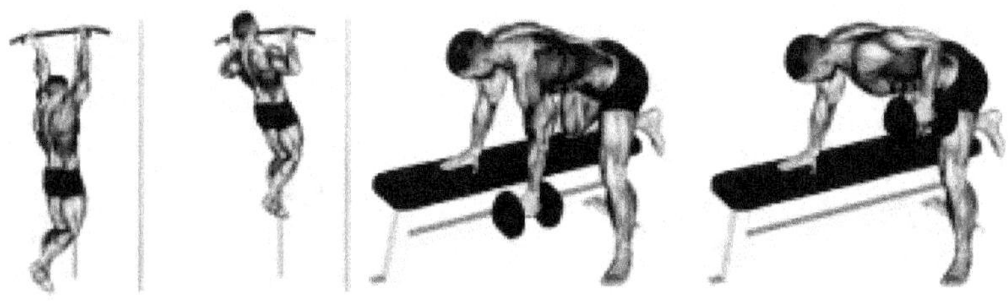

Barbell Bent Over Row

Cable Bar Lateral Pulldown

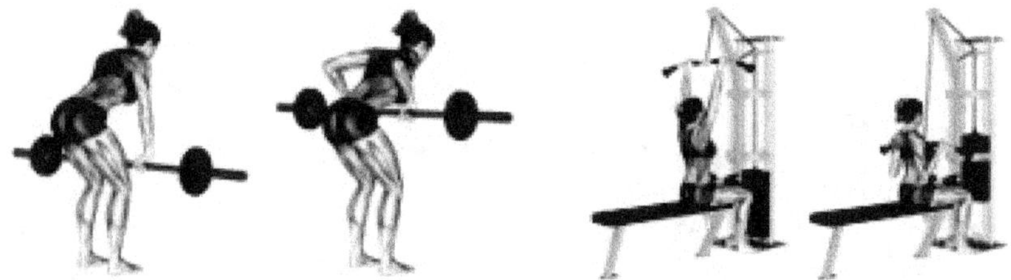

Legs

Barbell Dead Lift   Barbell Squat

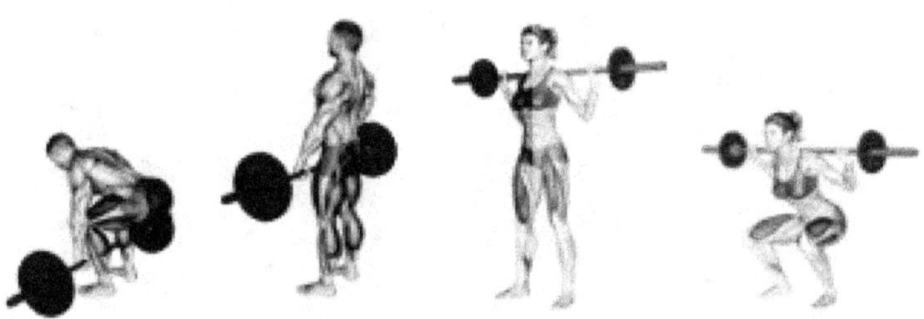

Dumbbell Forward Leaning Lunge   Dumbbell Squat

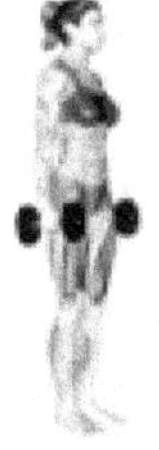
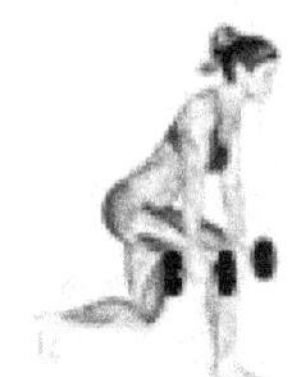
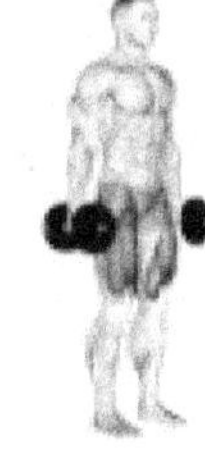
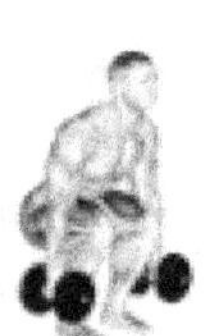

Dumbbell Dead Lift   Dumbbell Lunge with Bicep Curl

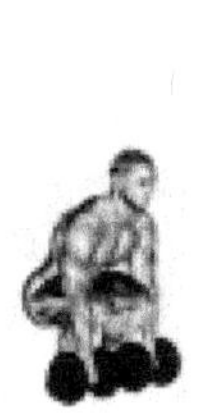
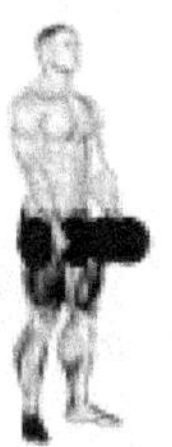
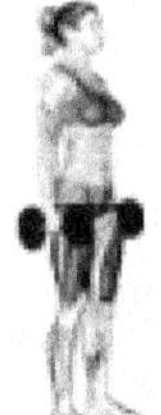
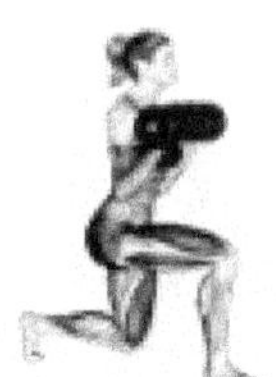

Summary

Hypertrophy
Faster Metabolism
Weight Loss
Anabolic State Zone
Sleep
Protein
Progressive Weight Training
No Stimulation
No Muscle Synthesis
Cortisol Production
No Change
No Change
No Change
Long Cardio Session
Catabolic State Zone
Desired Physique

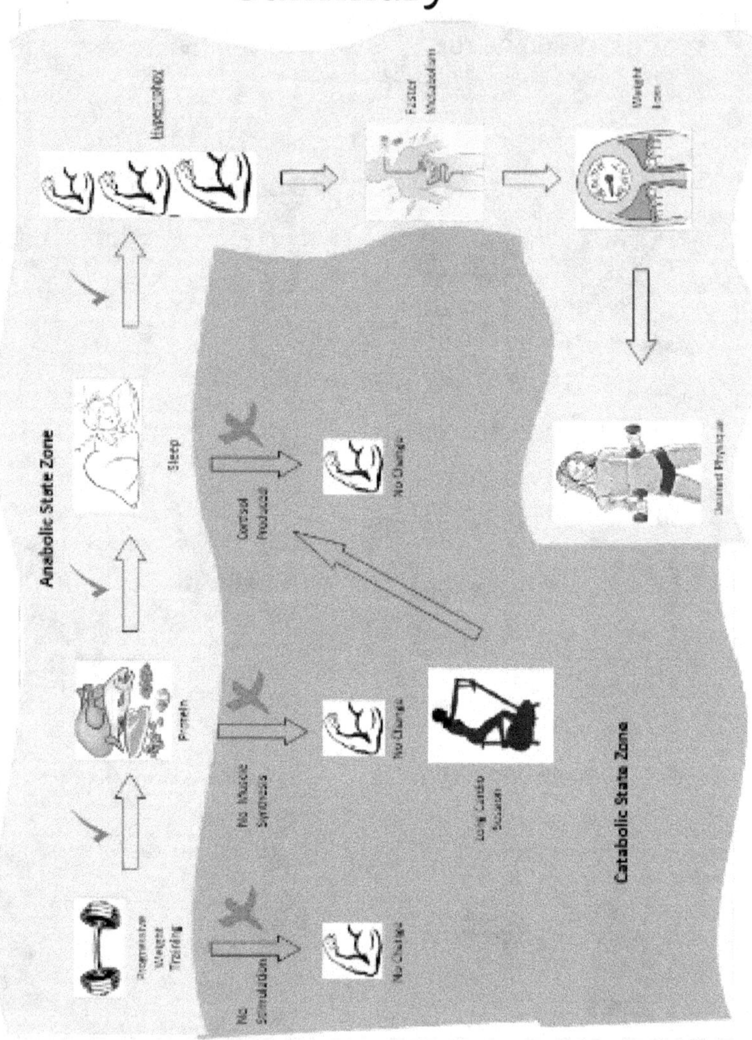

CHAPTER 14

Example Workouts:

When starting out, its best to start with mostly compound exercises that work multiple muscle groups and with perhaps 1 or 2 isolation exercises.

As previously said I recommend that you split your workouts into upper and lower body to allow enough time between workouts for recovery and muscle synthesis to take place.

Beginner: Routine 1 (2 Split)

Upper Body :

Chest

Barbell Bench Press	3 Sets 8 Reps 60% RM
Dumbbell Incline Press	3 Sets 8 Reps 60% RM

Shoulders

Dumbbell Shoulder Press	3 Sets 8 Reps 60% RM
Dumbbell Side Raise	3 Sets 8 Reps 60% RM

Back

Lat Pull Down	3 Sets 8 Reps 60% RM
Barbell Row	3 Sets 8 Reps 60% RM

Arms

EZ Bar Bicep Curl	3 Sets 8 Reps 60% RM
Cable Triceps Push Down	3 Sets 8 Reps 60% RM

Lower Body:

Legs

Seated Leg Curl	3 Sets 8 Reps 60% RM
Barbell Squats	3 Sets 8 Reps 60% RM
Leg Press	3 Sets8 Reps 60% RM
Dead Lift	3 Sets8 Reps 60% RM

Core

Plank	3 Sets 25 secs
Bench Leg Raises	3 Sets10 Reps
Ab Roller	3 Sets10 Reps

Beginner: Routine 2 (2 Split)

Upper Body :

Chest

Barbell Bench Press	3 Sets 8 Reps 60% RM
Dumbbell Incline Press	3 Sets 8 Reps 60% RM

Shoulders

Dumbbell Shoulder Press	3 Sets 8 Reps 60% RM
Dumbbell Front Raise	3 Sets 8 Reps 60% RM

Back

Lat Pull Down	3 Sets 8 Reps 60% RM
Dumbbell Row	3 Sets 8 Reps 60% RM

Arms

Dumbbell Bicep Curl	3 Sets 8 Reps 60% RM
Cable Triceps Push Down	3 Sets 8 Reps 60% RM

Lower Body:

Legs

Seated Leg Extension	3 Sets 8 Reps 60% RM
Kettle Bell Squats	3 Sets 8 Reps 60% RM
Lunges	3 Sets 8 Steps 60% RM
Dead Lift	3 Sets 8 Reps 60% RM

Core

Plank	3 Sets 25 secs
Bench Leg Raises	3 Sets 10 Reps
Ab Crunchies	3 Sets 10 Reps

It's very important that initially you concentrate on performing each exercise correctly. This ensures that the correct muscles are exercised and avoids possible injury.

After recovering from each routine, you can then start to increase the reps from 8 to 10 or 12 and you can start to add a little weight (1% - 5% increase until you reach around 75-85% of your 1 Rep Max (RM)). Keep doing this until you feel you can add a 4th Set. Only add weight if you can keep good form throughout the routine. Remember **good form trumps everything!**

As your fitness develops you can also start to reduce the rest periods between sets and different exercises.

Remember to keep a record of everything you've done (Gym Diary) and work towards progressing some part of your routine every time you work out.

Beginner: Routine 3
(after 12-16 weeks training) (2 Split)

Upper Body :

Chest

Barbell Bench Press	4 Sets 10 Reps 75-85% RM
Dumbbell Incline Press	4 Sets 10 Reps 75-85% RM
Dumbbell Chest Flys	4 Sets 10 Reps 75-85% RM

Shoulders

Dumbbell Shoulder Press	4 Sets 10 Reps 75-85% RM
Dumbbell Side Raise	4 Sets 10 Reps 75-85% RM
Dumbbell Front Raise	4 Sets 10 Reps 75-85% RM

Back

Lat Pull Down	4 Sets 10 Reps 75-85% RM
Barbell Row	4 Sets 10 Reps 75-85% RM

Arms

EZ Bar Bicep Curl	4 Sets 10 Reps 75-85% RM
Cable Triceps Push Down	4 Sets 10 Reps 75-85% RM
Dumbbell Triceps Kickback	4 Sets 10 Reps 75-85% RM

Lower Body:

Legs

Seated Leg Curl	4 Sets 10 Reps 75-85% RM
Seated Leg Extension	4 Sets 10 Reps 75-85% RM
Barbell Squats	4 Sets 10 Reps 75-85% RM
Leg Press	4 Sets 10 Reps 75-85% RM
Dead Lift	4 Sets 10 Reps 75-85% RM
Core Plank	4 Sets 60 secs
Bench Leg Raises	4 Sets 15 Reps
Ab Roller	4 Sets 15 Reps
Lateral Cable Twists	3 sets 12 Reps

These workouts are designed to be completed within approx. 60 mins. If it's taking you longer, then you are probably resting too much between sets or working too hard because your fitness and recovery aren't at that stage quite yet. A compound set is where you continue onto the next exercise without taking any rest. You can rest between compound sets, but it works even better if you don't.

Intermediate: Routine 1 Weeks (17 – 36) (3 Splits)

Upper Body Day 1 :

Chest

Barbell Bench Press	4 Sets 10 Reps 75-85% RM
Dumbbell Incline Press	4 Sets 10 Reps 75-85% RM
Dumbbell Cable Flys	4 Sets 10 Reps 75-85% RM
Dumbbell Bench Press	4 Sets 10 Reps 75-85% RM

Arms (Biceps)

EZ Bar Biceps Curl	4 Sets 10 Reps 75-85% RM
Dumbbell Biceps Curl	4 Sets 10 Reps 75-85% RM
Seated D/B Hammer Curls	4 Sets 10 Reps 75-85% RM
Neutral Grip Chin Ups	3 Sets 6 Reps

Abs

Crunchies	3 Sets 20 Reps
Cable Oblique Twists	3 Sets 12 Reps each side

Intermediate: Routine 1 Weeks (17 – 36) (3 Splits)

Upper Body Day 2 :

Shoulders

Dumbbell Shoulder Press	4 Sets 0 Reps 75-85% RM
Dumbbell Side Raise	4 Sets 10 Reps 75-85% RM
Dumbbell Front Raise	4 Sets 10 Reps 75-85% RM

Back

Lat Pull Down	4 Sets 10 Reps 75-85% RM
Barbell Row	4 Sets 10 Reps 75-85% RM

Arms

Cable Triceps Push Down	4 Sets 10 Reps 75-85% RM
Dumbbell Triceps Kickback	4 Sets 10 Reps 75-85% RM
EZ Bar Skull Crushers	4 Sets 10 Reps 75-85% RM

Lower Body Day 3:

Legs

Seated Leg Curl	4 Sets 10 Reps 75-85% RM
Seated Leg Extension	4 Sets 10 Reps 75-85% RM
Barbell Squats	4 Sets 10 Reps 75-85% RM
Leg Press	4 Sets 10 Reps 75-85% RM
Weighted Kettle Bell Lunges	4 Sets 16 Steps 60% RM

Core

Plank	4 Sets 70 secs
Bench Leg Raises	4 Sets 20 Reps
Ab Roller	4 Sets 20 Reps
Hollow Body Hold	3 sets 30 secs

When you first start these routines, it's possible you

may not quite reach the full number of sets or reps and that's ok. Just make that your goal and work towards achieving it (that counts as progression). But don't use very light weights to just achieve the reps. Better to start with a weight you can manage but feels like you are loading the muscle and then work towards getting the reps.

Remember that you build muscle when you are resting, not when you are exercising. The exercises are the stimulus for hypertrophy. Rest is when hypertrophy takes place.

These are only example routines and can be changed for other exercises that hit the same muscles but might be more suitable to the equipment that is available in your gym or at home. The splits can be done in any order as long as you ensure there is enough rest between each routine.

If you've got a smart phone, then Gymguide is a great app for selecting exercises. It gives you both images and short videos showing how each exercise should be done and a diagram showing which muscles will be targeted. The Garmin Connect app also offers something similar if you have one of their fitness watches.

One last thing never skip leg day, they are big muscles and offer the greatest return in your journey to raise your metabolism and lose that weight. They also offer the biggest gains in maintaining your mobility and avoiding fragility.

AFTERWORD

I'm glad you have made it this far and I do hope you have found this short book easy to read and informative. Now that you have enough of a basic understanding on how progressive resistance training works and the benefits it can bring to your weight control and general wellbeing. All you need to do now is get out to your local gym or get a home gym set up.

It's terrible that so few people know about the benefits of maintaining or building your lean tissue mass (muscle). A casual look at the average person on the street should confirm this to you.

It's not easy, and I never said it would be, but it's one hell of a lot easier, more healthy and more sustainable than restrictive diets (a battle that the majority of people never win).

Because it's based on energy expenditure (exercise), rather than energy intake (food), there's the added benefit of increasing your ability to do every day physical tasks. Walking upstairs is easy again. Imagine your new life to be active, not just when you go to the gym or do your workout for an hour. We all need to be more active throughout our daily lives. Perhaps there's the opportunity to take up an active pastime or sport that you never thought you could still do or just going for walks (with the added benefit of your increased lean body mass meaning that you get a greater fat burn for any given amount of exercise than the average person). Walking is low intensity and a great way to burn off some fat, as well as being a good time to listen to music or just meditate. The majority of the content in this book came to me whilst out walking.

Remember, because muscle takes time to build, it also takes time to get the results. In the early stages the results are less visibly noticeable, but underneath it is working, don't get despondent, keep going.

One last thing, success is based on progressing the resistance training. If you don't set your stall out to progress, then you won't progress. Remember that gym diary, so that you can record your workouts and see your progression. And remember, **good form trumps everything!** I really mean that. Irrespective of the weight used, if you don't do the exercise with good form, you won't get the results.

If you've enjoyed this book, found it informative and feel that others would benefit from my knowledge, would you mind taking a minute to leave an honest review on the amazon site where you made your purchase.

I'm always interested to hear if people enjoyed the knowledge I've shared with them and if there are any points that you feel I have missed, please let me know.

Now imagine you're in your 50s, but you can play like you are in your 30s!

Whatever your goals are, I know you can achieve them, so let your transformation begin and I wish you every success.

Good Luck!

Gavin

Note: *Whilst this book is about weight loss through progressive resistance training, I want to make it clear that I don't just do resistance training and I participate in other activities like cycling, HIIT and hill walking which keep me very active. However, I only achieved my ideal weight level through resistance training and managing my macros to suit my other activities.*

I like to eat and enjoy every calorie I've earned from my aerobic exercises.

ACKNOWLEDGMENTS

I'm sure this book would never have gone to print without the help from some of my friends.

I have to start by thanking Shannen Sneddon manager of my local gym (Burnawn Fitness) for taking an interest in my book and spending considerable amounts of her own time proof reading, making notes and highlighting areas that needed more explanation.

I would like to thank my friend Jan for becoming my rookie training partner and proving that starting from scratch and following my advice she could progress towards achieving the weight loss and body composition results she so much wanted. Well done Jan, it is a pleasure training with you and seeing your results steadily improve both within the gym and as a result, also for your cycling fitness. I'm sure others must notice the positive changes. However, I will also take this opportunity to apologise for the number of times you suffered DOMS as I introduced or tried different exercises within our routine and when we returned after 3 periods of lockdown. Sorry about that.

Also, my good friend Stuart for challenging some of the facts I were writing about and forcing me to do more research to back it up. This book probably wouldn't have materialised if it wasn't for him and I constantly debating the benefits of nutrition and exercise. His ability to out debate me on almost every occasion was the inspiration for this book. I had to find a way of being able to articulate better what I knew and wanted to say.

Also, my friend Anne for showing interest in the knowledge I was parting with and through further discussion with her, giving me the ideas on areas I needed to write about and also for her early proofreading.

Without the 4 Amigos regular group cycling trips and the regular group discussions over coffee and cake on this subject, this book would never have existed.

Thank you all.

References

[1]https://pubmed.ncbi.nlm.nih.gov/31121843/ Dietary Protein and Muscle Mass: Translating Science to Application and Health Benefit. 2019 May 22;11(5):1136. doi: 10.3390/nu11051136.

John W Carbone [1], Stefan M Pasiakos [2]

Affiliations expand

- PMID: 31121843
- PMCID: PMC6566799
- DOI: 10.3390/nu11051136

[2] Slowing bone loss with weight-bearing exercise - Harvard Health December 20, 2017Published: March, 2017

Slowing bone loss with weight-bearing exercise

[3] Hard Work Beats Talent When Talent Doesn't Work Hard (teamusa.org)

By Megan Bomba, USA Field Hockey Content Development Intern & Messiah College Student-Athlete | April 03, 2019, 2:19 p.m. (ET)

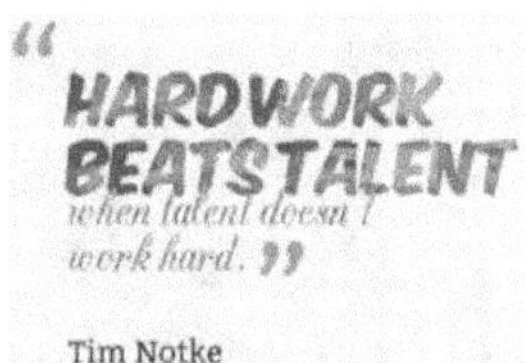

[4] Body type: Ben Creicos October 14, 2020

https://www.bodybuilding.com/fun/becker3.htm

[5] How Long Does it Take to Build Muscle and

BY   GAVIN TURNBULL

Increase Fat Loss? Florian Wuest December 16, 2020

[6] The Effects of Eating Too Many Carbs By Sylvie Tremblay, MSc Updated January 18, 2019

Gym Exercise Images are under a Royalty Free License from gymvisual.com and shutterstock.com

About the Author

Gavin Turnbull has lived in Ayrshire for over 20 years, although originally from the Borders. He has always had a passion for the outdoors and keeping fit enough to keep participating in the activities that he so much enjoys.

He has spent over 30 years weight training, road cycling, mountain biking, hill walking and generally spending large amounts of time being outdoors and active.

Now in his mid-fifties, he is more aware of how age changes our body composition and after extensive research and trial workouts has uncovered some of the basic facts and simple changes you can make to your lifestyle that can speed up your metabolism and get your body working like it was 20 years younger.

His key to keeping fit and active focuses on preventing muscle loss (sarcopenia), which in turn maintains a youthful metabolism allowing you to avoid restrictive diets and keep those energy levels up, along with all the other health benefits that resistance training offers.

Hopefully, this booklet will help others avoid the same mistakes he made on his journey to becoming leaner and fitter and achieve the same sustainable weight loss results he has.

www.ingramcontent.com/pod-product-compliance
Lightning Source LLC
Chambersburg PA
CBHW050737260726
48661CB00001B/282